THE TRUE HISTORY
OF THE ELEPHANT MAN

MICHAEL HOWELL AND PETER FORD

THE TRUE HISTORY OF THE ELEPHANT MAN

Revised and Illustrated Edition

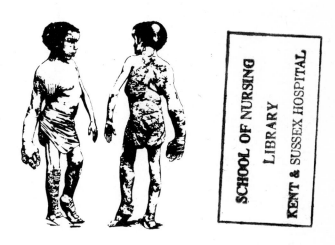

Allison & Busby
London & New York

First published 1980 by Allison & Busby Ltd,
6a Noel Street, London W1V 3RB
and distributed in the USA by Schocken Books Inc,
200 Madison Avenue, New York NY 10016 ·
Reprinted 1980, 1982

Revised and illustrated edition published 1983

Made and printed in Great Britain by
Butler & Tanner Ltd,
Frome and London

ISBN 0 85031 513 1

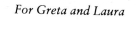

For Greta and Laura

CONTENTS

LIST OF PLATES

ACKNOWLEDGEMENTS

In reproducing the quotation from the journal which Lady Geraldine Somerset kept for the Duchess of Cambridge, we acknowledge the gracious permission of Her Majesty the Queen. We are also most grateful to Georgina Battiscombe, the biographer of Queen Alexandra, for drawing our attention to the existence of this reference in the Royal Archives, Windsor Castle Library, and to Sir Robin Mackworth-Young, the Librarian, for his help in supplying us with the text.

For permission to quote from the Minutes of the London Hospital House Committee, we are pleased to thank the London Hospital.

The book would hardly have been possible in its present form without the generous response of many individuals to what were often complex lines of inquiry. Above all, we have to thank Professor Gordon Seward of the London Hospital Medical College for the unstinted scope of his encouragement as well as for the time he has given to checking and making textual criticisms, especially of our final draft. J.P. Entract, former librarian of the London Hospital Medical College, and Percy Nunn, assistant curator of the college museum, have also been patient and more than helpful over a long period of time.

Others to whom we owe a special debt, both for kindness in general and for guiding us in the direction of much particular information, are W.J. Barlow; David Braithwaite; Colonel Rixon Bucknall, who helped to clarify the likely train ferry routes back to Harwich in 1886; G.W. Essex; Desmond Flower; E.R. Frizelle; John Garratt; Richard Carr-Gomm; Peter Honri; Mrs Leila Hoskins, for information about her aunt, Mrs Leila Maturin (née Leila Scot Skirving), and for providing us with a copy of the pamphlet printed as Appendix Two in this edition; Mrs Kenneth Lindy, daughter of Dr Tuckett, who also made available prints of the Elephant Man that had been among her father's papers; the London Library, for its facilities; the descendants of Tom Norman, and particularly Tom Norman Jnr, for making his unpublished memoirs available to us; Michael Pointon; Dr C.E. Taylor of Purley, who still possesses the chair which the Elephant Man used in the rooms which his grandfather, William Taylor, adapted for his use; Kate Thompson, archivist of the Leicester Museum, and the staff of the Leicester Museum and

Library; the descendants of Sam Torr, and especially Mrs Harry Heatherley (Patricia Torr), Mrs Hilda Metcalfe and Roy Torr, for placing their family collections of cuttings and memorabilia at our disposal; and Frederick Treves, great-nephew of Sir Frederick Treves, for his help and interest virtually since this search for the Elephant Man began.

Finally, we have to thank Margaret Robertson, who took new photographs for us in the London Hospital Medical College Museum; Dr Ron Finch, whose painstaking photographic skills made some excellent prints out of apparently unpromising archive material; and Pat Kingston, who, with the help of Janice Tipping, has handled the typing of successive drafts as well as much of the necessary correspondence.

ACKNOWLEDGEMENTS TO SECOND EDITION

New information on the background of Joseph Merrick's life has come to light since the original publication of this book and we have taken the opportunity of incorporating it into our revised text for this edition. In gathering this together, and for help with tracking down appropriate illustration material, we are grateful to the following:

Denis Clark has supplemented the work of Ron Finch in helping with photographs for this edition, and Curtis Lane & Co. of Sudbury, Suffolk, have given us an excellent service in the making of copy prints; Mrs Nellie Batchelor has been kind enough to tell us all she can remember of her uncle Walter Steel's recollections of having met Joseph Merrick; William Dooley (Benson Dulay) has generously told us not only about his uncle Sam Roper's fair, but has also passed on the family anecdotes as his late father, Bertram Dooley, recounted them about the time when he travelled with Joseph Merrick on the fairground circuits, and has made his family photographs available; Colin Eaton has unstintingly shared with us his researches in the Northamptonshire Records Office, drawing our attention to the presence there of Lady Louisa Knightley's diaries and putting us in touch with the families of Bertram Dooley and Walter Steel; the Great Eastern Railway Society has helped to supplement our earlier research, and we are especially grateful to Mr L.D. Brooks and Mr J. Sweiszkowski for steering us towards some rare picture material; Arthur Van Norman has helped us to round out the facts concerning the later part of the career of his father, Tom Norman; Nicholas Reed has given us access to the original Treves manuscript and kindly allowed us to consult the collection of Treves letters which he has in his possession; Julia Short has searched the photographic archives of the London Hospital for items for possible relevance; and Mr W.H. Steel has gone to some trouble to find and send us a surviving photograph of his father, Walter Steel.

CHAPTER 1

'The Great Freak of Nature
– Half-a-Man and Half-an-Elephant'

When the Elephant Man appeared as if from nowhere in a shop premises in the Whitechapel Road in London towards the end of November 1884, he was still in the early days of his career as a professional freak. His real name, as his birth certificate bears witness, was Joseph Carey Merrick, and his manager was Mr Tom Norman, a showman who specialized in the display of freaks and novelties. The shop hired for his exhibition was probably then numbered 123 Whitechapel Road. The building has survived until today as one in a terraced row of Victorian shops, though it has since been renumbered as 259. The adjoining premises on its east side carried the familiar pawnbroker's emblem of three iron balls high up on the wall. On the west side was the shop of Mr Michael Geary, fruiterer and greengrocer.

Directly across the road from the row of shops, on the other side of the wide thoroughfare, stands the imposing entrance to the London Hospital. The present front, however, dates from improvements made in 1891. In the 1880s the hospital displayed a long and imposing classical façade, set well back behind railings and with porters' lodges at the main gates. The whole effect was designed to inspire confidence in the capabilities of medical science, and no doubt a measure of appropriate awe among the inhabitants of the district. It was the outward and visible sign of authoritarian benevolence and charity in an area that had for many decades experienced an intimate connection with deprivation and poverty: one in which successive waves of penniless immigrants settled alongside the original communities of London's poor; those who, in the definition of the great Victorian pioneer in social investigation, Henry Mayhew, 'Will work, cannot work and will not work.'

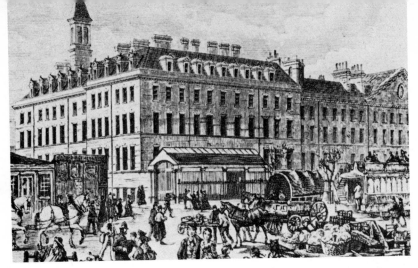

Plate 1. The front of the London Hospital as it was in 1876, showing the new Grocers' Wing to the left of the main façade (illustration from the *Illustrated London News*)

To such a district, then, Joseph Merrick was brought by Tom Norman, both of them hoping that the Elephant Man's impact on London would be profitable. Outside the premises, across the shop front, leaving only the doorway clear, the showman hung a large canvas sheet, painted with the startling image of a man half-way through the process of turning into an elephant and announcing that the same could be seen within for the entrance price of twopence. If the artistry was rough and its colours garish to sophisticated taste, the poster evidently had the sensational effect which the showman's skills intended. A young surgeon from the London Hospital, Mr Frederick Treves, who visited the freakshow, could recall the poster in all its vivid detail when he came to write about it some forty years later:

This very crude production depicted a frightful creature that could only have been possible in a nightmare. It was the figure of a man with the characteristics of an elephant. The transfiguration was not far advanced. There was still more of the man than of the beast. This fact – that it was still human – was the most repellent attribute of the creature. There was nothing about it of the pitiableness of the misshapened or the deformed, nothing of the grotesqueness of the freak, but merely the loathing insinuation of a man being changed into an animal. Some palm trees in the background of the picture suggested a jungle and might have led the imaginative to assume that it was in this wild that the perverted object had roamed.

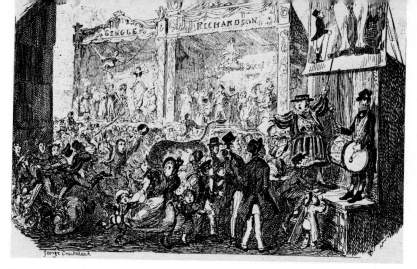

Plate 2. The hurly-burly of Bartholomew Fair depicted by George Cruikshank for his *Comic Almanack* (September 1835)

Whatever it was that could possibly be causing poor Merrick to take on his verisimilitude to an elephant, in displaying him as a freak Mr Norman was working in an ancient tradition which could trace its roots far back in the history of fairgrounds and circuses in England. London, in particular, had been noted for its insatiable appetite for monsters ever since at least the days of Elizabeth I. As Henry Morley stated in his *Memoirs of Bartholomew Fair*, it was not merely the common throng which sought out a formidable diet of signs and wonders and supported popular fashions in the grotesque. Everyone in society, up to the level of its crowned heads, 'shared in the tastes ... for men who could dance without legs, dwarfs, giants, hermaphrodites, or scaly boys'. He goes on to comment, writing his book in the late 1850s:

> The taste still lingers among uncultivated people in the highest and lowest ranks of life, but in the reign of William and Mary, or Queen Anne, it was almost universal. Bartholomew Fair, with all the prodigies exhibited therein, was not as it now would be, an annual display of things hardly to be seen out of a fair, but was, as far as Monsters went, only a yearly concentration into one spot of the entertainments that at other times were scattered over town and country.

Bartholomew Fair was officially opened each year on 23 August, the eve of Saint Bartholomew, and continued for two weeks. While the revels lasted, many poor tradesmen in the Smithfield area were glad to hire out a part of their premises for the display of some prodigy of nature. Prime sites were those shops or workrooms which were close to taverns, like the premises where a 'changeling child' could be viewed,

> next door to the *Black Raven* in West Smithfield ... being a living Skeleton, taken by a *Venetian* Galley, from a *Turkish* Vessel in the *Archipelago*. This is a Fairy Child, supposed to be born of *Hungarian* Parents, but chang'd in the Nursing, Aged Nine Years and more; not exceeding a foot and a half high. The Legs, Thighs and Arms are so very small, that they scarce exceed the bigness of a Man's Thumb, and the face no bigger than the Palm of one's hand.·

On another occasion, 'next door to the *Golden Hart* in *West-Smithfield*', there was to be seen 'the Admirable Work of Nature, a Woman having Three Breasts; and each of them affording Milk at one time, or differently, according as they are made use of'.

Advancing sharply up the social scale, the West End of London actually had its permanent exhibition halls available for hire to showmen. When, in 1826, the bookseller and radical pamphleteer William Hone interviewed Claude Amboise Seurat, the 'Anatomie Vivant; or Living Skeleton!' for the enlightenment of readers of his periodical journal *The Every-day Book*, he visited him in Pall Mall, in a room known as the Chinese Saloon. When

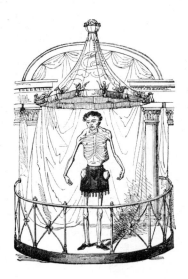

Plate 3. Claude Amboise Seurat, 'The Living Skeleton', on display in the Chinese Saloon in 1826 (from Hone's *Every-day Book*)

Barnum brought General Tom Thumb to London in 1844, the curiosity aroused was so phenomenal that he was able to engage the Egyptian Hall in Piccadilly. These remarkable premises were built in 1812 by William Bullock, to show his own vast and miscellaneous collection of curiosities, the nucleus for which he had gathered together during his earlier years as a silversmith in Liverpool when he bought rarities from sailors arriving at the port from exotic parts.

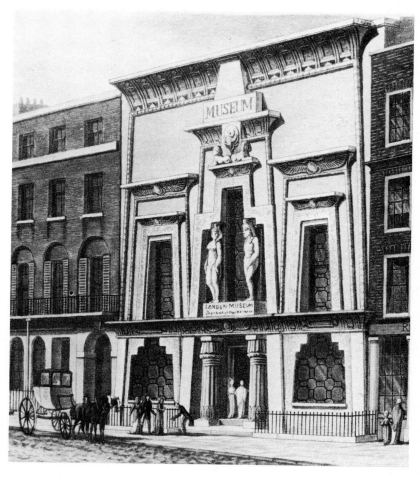

Plate 4. Bullock's Museum in Piccadilly, London, which later became known as the Egyptian Hall (reproduced from *Ackermann's Repository of Arts,* 1815)

The Egyptian Hall started life with cultural and educational pretensions, containing 'upwards of Fifteen Thousand Natural and Foreign Curiosities, Antiquities and Productions of the Fine Arts'. While these aspirations were never quite lost to sight, the lease passed into the hands of others and the Egyptian Hall became the recognized showplace for every nine-days' wonder that could be expected to excite a lively interest. Matters reached the pitch where *Punch*, in 1847, suggested the existence of an epidemic of a new disease

Plate 5. 'Deformito-mania': the taste for grotesque novelties is satirized in *Punch*, 4 September 1847

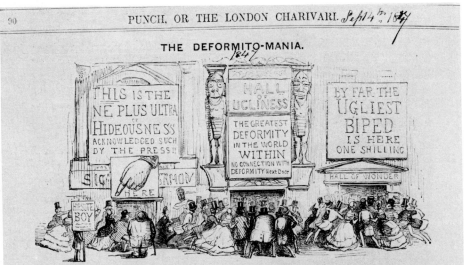

THE taste for the Monstrous seems, at last, to have reached its climax. The walls of the Egyptian Hall in Piccadilly are placarded from top to bottom with bills announcing the exhibition of some frightful object within, and the building itself will soon be known as the Hall of Ugliness. We cannot understand the cause of the now prevailing taste for deformity, which seems to grow by what it feeds upon. The first dose administered to this morbid appetite was somewhat homœopathic, being comprised in the diminutive form of TOM THUMB; but the eagerness with which this little humbug was devoured—at least by female kisses—has caused the importation, on a much larger scale, of all sorts of *lusus naturæ* and specimens of animated ugliness, which form a source of attraction to the public, and are exhibited with success in the very building where HAYDON in vain invited attention to the creations of his genius.

If *Beauty and the Beast* should be brought into competition in London, at the present day, *Beauty* would stand no chance against the *Beast* in the race for popularity. We understand that an exhibition consisting of the most frightful objects in nature is about to be formed at the Egyptian Hall, under the now taking title of the Hideorama. Poor MADAME TUSSAUD, with her Chamber of Horrors, is quite thrown into the shade by the number of real enormities and deformities that are now to be seen, as the showmen say, "Alive! alive!" Her wax is snuffed out, or extinguished, by the new lights now shining in Piccadilly, where a sort of Reign of Terror just now prevails.

There seems to be a sort of fascination in the horrible; and we can only hope, as the mania has now reached its extreme, a healthy admiration for the "true and the beautiful," as the novelists call it, will immediately begin to show itself.

termed 'Deformito-mania' and published a cartoon satirizing the placards decorating the Egyptian Hall's façade.

It is a long walk from the West End to Whitechapel; but appropriately enough the route from Smithfield can be retraced back along Cheapside, through the City of London and eventually along the Whitechapel Road – appropriately, since this was the main route into London from East Anglia and the Eastern Counties. It was the route taken by the drovers who walked herds of cattle for sale at Smithfield market to keep the metropolis supplied with fresh meat. The Whitechapel Road is still part of the main thoroughfare into central London for traffic from the east, and its exceptional width is a legacy of its origins as a droving road. It is this width, in turn, which has made it a natural location for the street market traders' stalls which continue to do business there, if no longer in the colourful profusion that must have set the scene during the late nineteenth century.

There was another young surgeon who stumbled across the Elephant Man in his original London exhibition even earlier than Frederick Treves. John Bland-Sutton, from the Middlesex Hospital, was in later years to become a consulting surgeon to the Middlesex Hospital, President of the Royal College of Surgeons, and a baronet, but in 1884 he had only just attained his fellowship of the Royal College of Surgeons. As he recorded in his collection of autobiographical reminiscences, *The Story of a Surgeon*, he was in the habit of wandering out through the East End of London as far as the Mile End Road to satisfy a mixture of professional interest and idle curiosity:

> ... especially on Saturday nights, to see dwarfs, giants, fat-women, and monstrosities at the freak shows. There was a freak-museum at a public-house – The Bell and Mackerel, near the London Hospital. It was on one of these visits in 1884 I saw 'on show' opposite the London Hospital a repulsive human being known as the Elephant Man. The poor fellow, John [sic] Merrick – was deformed in body, face, head and limbs. His skin, thick and pendulous, hung in folds and resembled the hide of an elephant – hence his show-name.

In another autobiography, *A Labrador Doctor*, Sir Wilfred Grenfell, whose early medical training was gained at the London Hospital, made the suggestion that it was some medical students from the hospital who first went to view the Elephant Man in the exhibition shop, and then returned to describe him to their surgeon-lecturer in anatomy, Frederick Treves. Certainly in his unpublished memoirs, the showman himself, Mr Tom Norman, remembered how

> ... there was, every week-day, morning and afternoon up till about 3 p.m. a number of students with white coats and no hats, passing in and out of the London Hospital opposite for the purpose of which I then presumed to obtain refreshments, fresh air, etc. After a few had,

out of curiosity visited the exhibition, the wonderful sight of Meyrick [*sic*] soon spread amongst them, and no doubt that is the reason of Sir Frederick's visit.

In fact, it was Frederick Treves's house surgeon who first told him about the Elephant Man. Dr Reginald Tuckett was then twenty-four years old and employed by the hospital in the most junior of its appointments. He had begun his medical studies as an articled pupil to his brother-in-law, a doctor in the Welsh border country. To qualify for admission to the Medical Register, however, he had come to the London Hospital to complete his training. It was now a little more than a year since he qualified, and he was employed by the hospital as house physician, house surgeon and resident accoucheur. But the burden of his responsibilities did not prevent his being enticed across the road by the showman's poster. The graphic account of the exhibit that he carried back to the hospital was compelling enough to prompt Treves into making his own pilgrimage to the north side of the Whitechapel Road to view the Elephant Man.

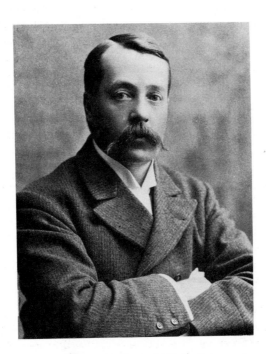

Plate 6. Dr Reginald Tuckett

When he arrived outside the shop it was to find the exhibition temporarily closed. Questioning a small boy hanging about on the pavement revealed where the showman might be found, and the lad was persuaded to seek him out, where he was refreshing himself in one of the local taverns. Mr Tom Norman proved unhesitating when it came to striking a bargain: he would open the exhibition for a private view, on condition that the special entrance fee of one shilling was paid. The scene was set for Frederick Treves's first encounter with Joseph Merrick, the Elephant Man.

The classic account of that meeting is contained in the title essay of *The Elephant Man and Other Reminiscences*. It is reproduced in its full text as the third appendix of the present book (pages 230–46). Within a well-told anecdote, Treves presents a series of vivid images; it is a powerful and unforgettable literary achievement. It may rest a little heavily on melodrama, but it remains as highly readable as when it was written, and fully deserves to be read. On the other hand, it raises incidental questions about the relationship between objective truth and the validity of literary creation, and should not be looked at uncritically.

Treves was certainly not starting out to write fiction when, towards the end of his life, he finally set down the tale of the Elephant Man for inclusion in what was to be his last published work. His essay, however, is not strictly factual. There are errors of detail: the London Hospital does not stand in the Mile End Road, as he states in the opening sentence. There are numerous indications of how over the years his memory became overlaid with small, embellishing details that undeniably add colour and effect to the story-telling. Above all, there is the curious fact that he consistently saddles Joseph Merrick with the Christian name of John. It seems curious, because a whole segment of Treves's life and career came to be intertwined with the destiny of Joseph Merrick, and, as things turned out, it was hardly a superficial relationship.

Could it have been that the facial distortions which were a part of Merrick's condition, and which made comprehensible speech extremely difficult for him, meant that Treves misheard? Was it possible that Treves heard 'Joseph' as 'John' during the course of an early conversation and so ever afterwards thought of him as and called him 'John'? On the other hand, others heard and recorded his name correctly. It was unlikely that it could have been simply a loss of memory. From the very beginning of their relationship Treves was writing of Merrick as 'John'. Did Merrick himself prefer the name? Evidently not, for he called himself Joseph and signed himself Joseph in a surviving letter (page 143). By this stage these can be no more than speculations, and only recently has a further clue come to the surface to enlighten the mystery (see page 213). Yet Treves's misnomer as applied to Merrick has had one long-term side-effect: almost every reference to the Elephant Man printed since has repeated the error because the authors cannot believe that Treves got such a basic detail wrong.

One other minor discrepancy concerns the identity of the shop where Mr Tom Norman set up his exhibition. It was, says Treves, 'a vacant green-grocer's which was to let'. He goes on to sketch in a few scenic props:

> The shop was empty and grey with dust. Some old tins and a few shrivelled potatoes occupied a shelf and some vague vegetable refuse the window.

Yet Tom Norman was stung into writing an emphatic letter to the press when he first heard about Treves's essay, and among the details that he wished to correct was the fact that Merrick 'was not exhibited in an empty greengrocer's shop'.

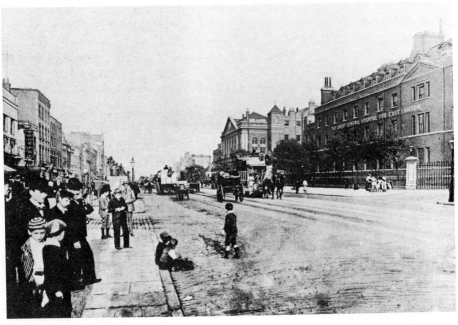

Plate 7. The broad highway of the Whitechapel Road outside the London Hospital. The shop in which the Elephant Man was displayed was directly opposite the main entrance (reproduced from *Round London*, 1896)

That shop [he says] was next door to the one he was exhibited in, and kept by a man named Geary, an Irishman in the Whitechapel Road. The shop on the other side of the one we were showing was ... a pawnbroker's. The premises used for the exhibition of Meyrick [*sic*] had for several years previously been a waxworks museum owned by a man of the name of Cotton. I came to London and rented it from him, and removed Meyrick thereto.

According to the *London Directory* for 1886, prepared in 1885, the greengrocer's shop opposite to the London Hospital was, indeed, kept by a Mr Michael Geary. It appears that he took possession of his shop towards the end of 1884, for the directory prepared in that year lists the occupier as a Mr William Parry. Next door but one to the greengrocer's there was also, indeed, the pawnbroker's. The shop premises at 123 Whitechapel Road, now 259, sandwiched between the pawnshop and the fruiterer's, is recorded in the directories as a glass warehouse belonging to Albert and Eli Shepherd. In view of Tom Norman's precise statement and the corroborative evidence from the directories, it seems reasonable to accept that it was the front portion of this shop which was sub-let to Mr Cotton for use as a waxworks museum. There can be no doubt that a waxworks museum did flourish opposite to the London Hospital, for in September 1888, in the midst of the Whitechapel murders committed by 'Jack the Ripper', a correspondent who called himself John Law was writing in the columns of the *Pall Mall Gazette*:

There is at present almost opposite the London Hospital a ghastly display of the unfortunate woman murdered ... An old man exhibits these things, and while he points them out you will be tightly wedged in between a number of boys and girls, while a smell of death rises into your nostrils, and you feel as if your throat was filled up with fungus.

It therefore seems reasonably certain that it was the door of 123 Whitechapel Road which Mr Tom Norman in due course unlocked and opened, before ushering his visitor from the hospital opposite into the dark interior.

It was difficult for the visitor to pick out anything at first, for the light from the window was obstructed by the large canvas sheet bearing its message to the passers-by in the street. The atmosphere was decidedly cold and damp, and there was a faint but peculiarly unpleasant odour hanging in the air. The main part of the shop was bare and disused, but towards the back a cord had been suspended across the room from one side to the other, and what might have been a large red tablecloth hung down from it to form an improvised screen.

As soon as they were in the shop, Tom Norman went across to the screen and drew it aside. There, in the half-light beyond, sat the figure of the Elephant Man, seemingly remarkably small in contrast to the impression of something gigantic created by the showman's poster. He was hunched up upon a stool, and held a brown blanket drawn well up about himself to cover his head and shoulders. The movement of the curtain did not seem to disturb him, for he continued to sit motionless, staring at the blue flame of a gas burner arranged so as to heat a large brick balanced on a tripod before him. This was the only source of heat and light in the room. The very stillness of the almost diminutive figure awoke in Treves the feeling, as he said, that here was the very 'embodiment of loneliness'.

The showman suddenly called out a sharp instruction to the figure: 'Stand up!' Treves says that he spoke 'harshly', 'as if to a dog', implying a brutal insensitivity on the part of the Elephant Man's keeper. Yet Mr Norman was a professional in his own area, and how else would his public expect him to behave when dealing with a creature supposedly half-human, half-beast – a kind of urban Caliban?

But then, as if reluctantly, the Elephant Man stirred and rose awkwardly to his feet, letting the blanket slip to the ground as he turned to face this most exclusive audience. As the covering fell, the source of the peculiar odour which hung in the air inside the shop became apparent, for the sickening stench, which evidently had its origins in the startling condition of the subject's body, at once intensified.

Treves's medical career had been associated with the London Hospital from the beginning. He had arrived as a medical student in 1871, become assistant surgeon at the hospital in 1879, and was appointed full surgeon there in 1884. Although he was still only thirty-one, his experience of the appalling range of physical horrors and injuries likely to be admitted into a foundation which existed to minister to the ills of an area which contained some of the worst slums of Europe must have been considerable. It would therefore be reasonable to expect him to be shock-proof, his nose used to such smells as that of gangrene, his eyes accustomed, for example, to the terrible facial injuries which could result from a fight with broken bottles in any London pub on a Saturday night. From what he says, however, it is clear that he was shaken by his first glimpse of Joseph Merrick; and perhaps also taken unawares by his revulsion at the sickening stench given off by Merrick's body. He summed up his initial reaction in one memorable phrase: that Merrick seemed to him 'the most disgusting specimen of humanity'. 'At no time,' wrote Treves, 'had I met with such a degraded or perverted version of a human being as this lone figure displayed.'

As he stared, the Elephant Man began to turn slowly about so that his visitor might view him from all angles. The movement re-awakened Treves's clinical instincts, for he noticed how the unfortunate creature showed signs of having at some time in life suffered a disease of the left hip; it had left him lame so that he needed to lean on a stick. With the return of his habit of scientific detachment, Treves began to make precise clinical observations. Where he had been expecting to see a figure that was both monstrous and large, the Elephant Man was in fact of quite a slight build, perhaps only a little over five foot two inches in height. The upper part of his body was unclothed to the waist, and the lower half was clad in a pair of threadbare trousers that seemed to have 'once belonged to some fat gentleman's dress suit'. The feet were also naked, and his lameness became obvious as he stood there with his body slightly tilted to the left and his back twisted and bent.

Above all, it was the head which created such an amazing impression. This did indeed seem huge beyond Treves's most imaginative expectations: a misshapen mass of bony lumps and cauliflower-like growths of skin. It had the circumference of a man's waist, and the forehead was disfigured by bosses of bony material which bulged forward in great mounds, giving it an appearance something like that of a cottage loaf laid on its side. The greater mound pressed down upon the right eyebrow so that the eye on that side of the skull was almost hidden.

The lower half of the face was itself compressed and distorted by a swelling of the right cheek, where a pink mass of flesh protruded from the mouth, forcing back the lips into inverted folds. Here, then, was the origin of the 'trunk' which the poster artist had so graphically portrayed, if with a certain artistic licence to enhance its resemblance to an elephant's anatomy. There were other bony masses present on the top and side of the skull, but in those areas it was the skin which dominated, the flesh being raised up into heavy cauliflower-textured growths that hung down at the sides and back of the head.

Merrick's body itself was in no way spared, for masses of similar pendulous growths of skin hung down from the chest and back. Elsewhere it looked as though the skin was covered by fine warts. The right arm was enormous in size and virtually shapeless, the hand on that side being 'large and clumsy – a fin or paddle rather than a hand ... The thumb had the appearance of a radish, while the fingers might have been thick tuberous roots.' It was impossible to imagine such a limb being of much use to its owner. By contrast, the left arm and hand looked completely normal, even delicate and feminine in their refinement. The feet, so far as Treves could see, were as shapeless and deformed as the gross right arm.

The showman seemed to Treves to be unable or reluctant to pass on more than the most rudimentary information about his charge: that he was English born, that he was twenty-one years old and that his name, so Treves states him as saying, was John Merrick. For his own part, Treves felt a keen perplexity in the face of the malformations which he found himself observing. He was certainly quite unable to account for the condition, to pin on it any label of medical diagnosis or to recall ever having come across anything remotely like it in his professional experience or theoretical training.

Treves was already a figure to be reckoned with in the medical world. In 1881 he had been invited by the Royal College of Surgeons to give the Erasmus Wilson Lectures, a series of six lecture-demonstrations on specimens from the college's museum to be delivered before an audience consisting of some of the most distinguished surgeons in the country. He added to this honour the winning of the college's Jacksonian Prize in 1883 for an original essay on intestinal surgery. In the same year he published *Surgical Applied Anatomy*, a textbook which lost no time in establishing itself as both a standard reference work and a medical best-seller. If he was disconcerted or discomforted by his bewilderment on viewing the sorely afflicted frame of Joseph Merrick, he must have been stimulated by the challenge which it presented to his diagnostic abilities and to his natural instincts as a scientific investigator.

The explanation which Mr Norman offered to account for his protégé's deformities at least had the advantage of simplicity. All this came about, the showman explained, as the consequence of an unfortunate accident. While the Elephant Man's mother was carrying him during the last few months of her pregnancy, she was knocked over and badly frightened by an elephant from a travelling menagerie. The shock thus sustained conveyed itself to the unborn child, with the result which they saw before them. Dr Bland-Sutton also remembered having heard this story in connection with his visit to the freakshow, so it may be taken as an integral part of the showman's patter. As will be seen later, Merrick himself clung to this story, finding in it a strange degree of comfort. By implication, the extreme rarity of his sensational disorder could no doubt be accounted for by the scarcity of runaway elephants in rural England.

Frederick Treves's interest in the case, however, was not concerned with exploring it as medical folk-belief. Rather than the vagaries of superstition, his instincts were to seek to establish scientific fact and, if appropriate, write up an account of these apparently undescribed abnormalities for publication. His mind was quite made up by now that he would like to take Merrick back across the road so that he could examine him at leisure and in detail in his room in the London Hospital's Medical College. Mr Norman once more proved willing to strike a bargain, for no doubt he saw a publicity value in this idea. It was therefore agreed. But then, wrote Treves, 'I became at once conscious of a difficulty.'

Considerable problems must invariably have been involved in transporting this startling being about from place to place. The problem, moreover, still existed, even when moving him over a distance of no more than a few hundred yards to the door of the Medical College, which lay along Turner Street, on the south-west side of the London Hospital's main complex of buildings. For the Elephant Man to appear on the streets without concealment was, in fact, to invite the immediate assembling of an unruly crowd. In the open, out of his refuge, Merrick's footsteps had invariably been dogged by an ever-increasing excitement and clamour, his progress hampered by eager, curious, shocked and frankly incredulous bystanders. Mr Norman, it can be assumed, took relish in cataloguing the dramatic effects which his charge was capable of launching on the Queen's Highway. The Elephant Man's journeyings abroad were, it seemed, in the habit of degenerating into public disturbances.

There was nevertheless a solution to hand – or, at least, a partial solution. It took the form of a special set of outdoor clothes which the Elephant Man possessed and could use to conceal himself from head to toe. The whole outfit consisted of three garments. First there came a pair of huge, bag-like slippers in which the feet and lower legs could be encased. Then there was the voluminous black cloak which practically touched the ground once it was draped round its owner's shoulders. Treves could only remember having seen such a garment once before, and then it had been at a play in the theatre, when it was 'wrapped about the figure of a Venetian bravo'. He found it difficult to imagine how the Elephant Man could ever have come by such a garment, but the most extraordinary item of clothing remained the hat. This was shaped somewhat like a conventional peaked cap, and was also black in colour. Its dimensions, however, were vast, since it naturally needed to be large enough to fit over the Elephant Man's head. From the edge of the wide peak a brownish flannel pelmet hung down to conceal the face, but in this a horizontal slit was cut so that Merrick could see where he was going.

As Treves remarked, the sight of the Elephant Man limping slowly along in his outdoor clothing – a slight, bent figure, leaning heavily upon a stick and engulfed in a huge black cloak, the whole ensemble topped off by the great heavy head in its 'pillar-box' hat – could have been only a degree or two less alarming than the appearance of the man unclothed. It was eventually agreed

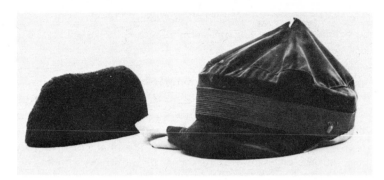

Plate 8. The Elephant Man's 'pillar-box' hat (a), and (b) the hat and pelmet on the cast of his head in the London Hospital

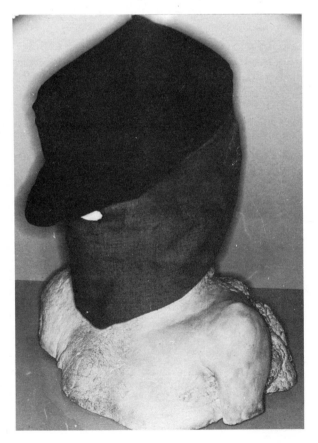

that Merrick would wear outdoor garments for his visit to the Medical School, but that Treves would hire a cab to carry him from door to door and return him in the same way afterwards.

There remained only the need to ensure the smooth reception of the Elephant Man at the college. So that he might identify himself to the porter and avoid any embarrassing delays at the entrance, Treves handed Merrick his visiting card. The first meeting between Frederick Treves, a young surgeon with an ever more ambitious career before him, and Joseph Merrick, the Elephant Man, a humble freak whose hopes for the future were of an altogether more modest character, was over.

CHAPTER 2

On the Threshold of Eminence

By any standards, Treves cut an impressive figure. Indeed, he might almost have posed for a monument to what it was possible to achieve by a combination of a peculiarly Victorian trio of virtues: industry, tenacity and talent. He had reached the age of thirty-one with his life already a success story.

Treves was a Dorset man, from the county town of Dorchester, the youngest son in the family of William Treves, a well-to-do furniture salesman and upholsterer. William Treves kept a large town house above his shop, which stood in one of the main streets of the town. It was there, at 8 Cornhill, Dorchester, on 15 February 1853, that Frederick Treves was born.

Little is recorded of his early life. At the age of seven his education began at the small Dorchester school where his brothers had been taught before him. The headmaster of the school was the Reverend William Barnes (1801–86), a formidable scholar and linguist who was nevertheless also a dialect poet of sensitivity and an important influence in English literary history. Both Gerard Manley Hopkins and Thomas Hardy acknowledged a debt to his influence in their poetry.

When he was writing the Dorset volume for the *Highways and Byways* topographical series on the English counties, Treves remembered the extraordinary range of his old master:

> He was familiar with all European languages ... He could read Hindustani, Persian, Arabic and other unwonted tongues. He was a very accomplished musician, playing himself the flute, the violin, and the piano. He wrote innumerable books besides his well-known poems,

and was learned in geology and archaeology. More curious still, he was a competent engraver on both wood and copper, so that he illustrated not only his own works ... but also the books and monographs of his friends.

Treves was only at William Barnes's school for two years, but the impression left on him by this Dorset genius, who managed to combine an austere and rigorous regard for learning with a broad humanity and a delicacy of vision, was clearly life-long. When he entered school, Treves told his publisher, Newman Flower, many years later, he 'was very frightened by the austere figure in black, sitting there like some grim Inquisitor in the high chair'. Mary Hardy, Thomas Hardy's younger sister who was also a pupil at the school, remembered Treves as a shy and even timid child who would, the moment school was over, run to hide in the cloakroom behind the coats of the other pupils until the family maid came to escort him home. Despite all this, Treves wrote that his recollection of Barnes was:

> ... that of the gentlest and most kindly of men. His appearance was peculiar. He had white hair and a long white beard, and always wore knee breeches and shoes with large buckles. Out of doors he donned a curious cap and a still more curious cape, while I never saw him without a bag over his shoulder and a stout staff. During school hours he was in the habit of pacing the room in a reverie, happily oblivious of his dull surroundings. I remember once that some forbidden fruit of which I was possessed rolled across the schoolroom floor, and that I crawled after it in the wake of the dreaming master. He turned suddenly in his walk and stumbled over me, to my intense alarm. When he regained his balance he apologized very earnestly and resumed his walk, unconscious that the object he had fallen over was a scholar. I have often wondered to which of his charming poems I owed my escape from punishment.

In due course, when he was eleven, Treves was sent to London, where his father had enrolled him at the Merchant Taylors' School. He stayed at Merchant Taylors' until he was eighteen, but as a scholar he seems to have left an undistinguished record. It was only in sports, and in football in particular, that he excelled, and holidays were always a time of happy return to his home county. Throughout his later life he was to speak with deep nostalgia of what he called 'the Dorset beyond the hills'.

It was decided eventually that he should follow his eldest brother, who had been a medical student at St Thomas's Hospital, into the medical profession. For the youngest Treves boy, though, a place was sought at the

Medical School attached to the London Hospital. It was perhaps a surprising choice. Of all the hospitals in London which then had medical schools attached to them, the London Hospital was generally considered the least attractive.

Plate 9. A typical back-street scene in Victorian Whitechapel: Brick Lane market (reproduced from *Round London*, 1896)

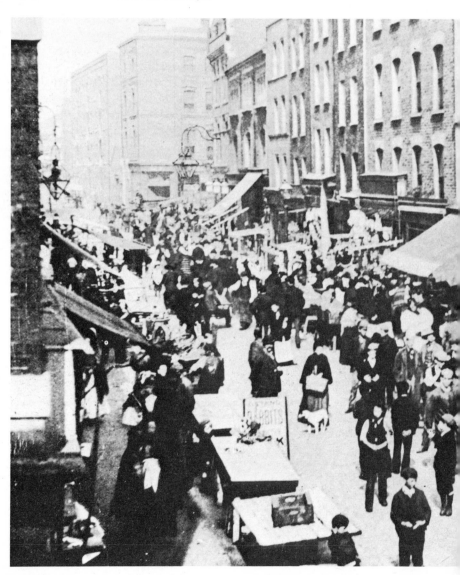

First and foremost there was the matter of its geographical situation. While it could claim at this time to be the largest hospital in England, it was set in the midst of the poorest population in the country. Its 690 beds drew patients from a maze of alleys, courts and back streets which stretched along the river behind the wharfs and docks of the lower Thames. It was, after all, *the* hospital of London's East End. Patients would arrive on handcarts from the markets of Billingsgate, on stretchers from as far away as Tilbury Docks

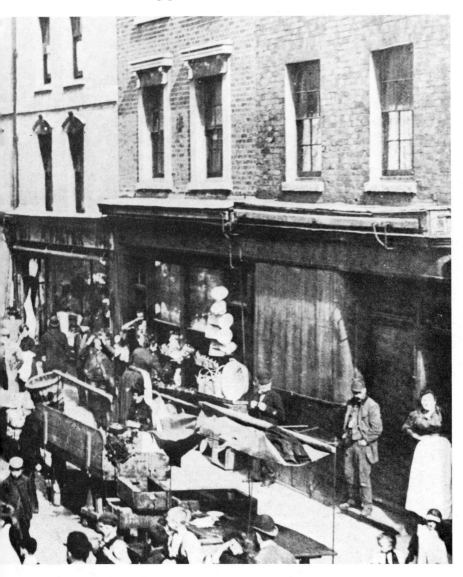

and from every noisome, rat-infested slum between the two. The poverty of the area, the overcrowding and filth, were almost indescribable. Portman Square off Orchard Street, for example, was a small court twenty-two feet wide with a common sewer running down the middle. Yet it served twenty-six three-storeyed houses and almost a thousand people regarded the square as home. In Wapping, the courtyards were deep in filth, and the children, often practically naked, would crawl to search for vegetable parings in the refuse. The Thames itself, which had become the great sewer for the entire metropolis, was so offensive that Members of Parliament at Westminster complained they could not use the room overlooking the river.

The London Hospital could doubtless claim that it had no shortage of good clinical material, but it was still hardly surprising if many students coming down from Oxford or Cambridge preferred to go to some other hospital to complete their studies. If the surroundings were depressing, however, the clinical teaching was superb. The teachers included such men as Jonathan Hutchinson, a tall, bearded surgeon who excelled in every field of medicine and who made so many original observations that his name is still to be found in modern textbooks of surgery; Hughlings Jackson, a brilliant and eccentric physician who has come to be recognized as one of the founders of neurology; Langdon Down, a specialist in the problems of mental deficiency who first recognized the existence of mongolism (now known more correctly as Down's syndrome) as an entity; and Andrew Clark, a doctor remembered not so much for his contributions to medical science as for the fact that he was chosen as personal physician by members of the Royal Family and by the Liberal prime minister, W.E. Gladstone. The young Robert Louis Stevenson travelled from Edinburgh to London to consult Clark about the condition of his tubercular lungs.

For the students, work at the London seems to have been haphazard and largely unsupervised, but its basis was unremittingly practical. Their help was necessary to cope with the scrimmage of patients who came in through the hospital doors like a tide continually on the flood. In 'The Old Receiving Room', a companion essay to 'The Elephant Man', Treves left a series of vivid vignettes of the mêlée of human distress which could develop in the casualty department in the days when he was a student, when the cry to go up in the event of an accident in the London streets was not yet, 'Call for an ambulance!' but still, 'Send for a shutter!'

The receiving unit consisted first of the hall, which served as waiting room and where there was always someone waiting:

It may be a suffering woman who has called for her dead husband's clothes. It may be a still breathless messenger with a 'midwifery card' in her hand, or a girl waiting for a dose of emergency medicine. There may be some minor accident cases also, such as a torn finger, or a black eye like a bursting plum, a child who has swallowed a halfpenny, and a woman who has been 'knocked about cruel', but has little to show for it except a noisy desire to have her husband 'locked up'.

Then, on each side of the hall, were two dressing-rooms, assigned respectively to men and women, where surgeons and dressers worked on the emergencies on a wide couch, sinisterly covered in thick, black and much-washed leather.

It may be a man ridden over in the street with the red bone-ends of his broken legs sticking through his trousers. It may be a machine accident, where strips of cotton shirt have become entangled up with torn flesh and a trail of black grease. It may be a man picked up in a lane with his throat cut, or a woman, dripping foul mud, who has been dragged out of the river.

Finally, there were the solemnly silent processions which accompanied every street casualty all the way to the hospital gates in the days before the introduction of ambulances, any diversion from life's hard routine no doubt being something to be made more than welcome.

It is a closely packed crowd which moves like a clot, which occupies the whole pavement and oozes over into the road. In the centre of the mass is an obscure object towards which all eyes are directed. In the procession are many women, mostly with tousled heads, men, mostly without caps, a butcher, a barber's assistant, a trim postman, a white-washer, a man in a tall hat, and a pattering fringe of ragged boys ...

The object carried would be indistinct, being hidden from view as is the queen bee in a clump of fussing bees. Very often the injured person is merely carried along by hand, like a parcel that is coming to pieces. There would be a man to each leg and to each arm, while men on either side would hang on to the coat. Possibly some Samaritan, walking backwards, would help hold up the dangling head. It was a much prized distinction to clutch even a fragment of the sufferer or to carry his hat or the tools he had dropped.

Plate 10 (overleaf). Sketches from a London hospital, reproduced from the *Graphic*, 27 December 1879

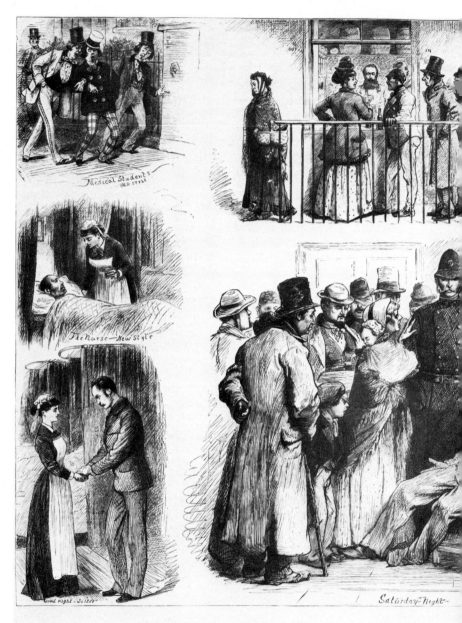

Medical Students *old style*

The Nurse—*New Style*

Good night—*Sister*

Saturday-Night

NOTES AT A

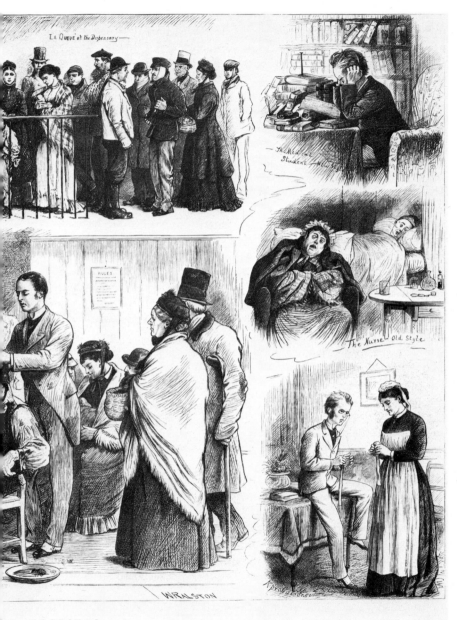

THE QUEUE at the Dispensary —

The Medical Student at Work

The Nurse — Old Style

A Probationer

W.RALSTON

ON HOSPITAL

In fact the busy unsupervised atmosphere at the London Hospital seems to have suited Treves exactly, and he began to display a determinedly practical approach to the problems he encountered. The firm decisions and decisive actions inherent in the surgical approach to patients seemed ideally suited to his personality, and it was to this branch of medicine that he found himself increasingly attracted.

After four years at the London Hospital, Treves's studies were completed, and in 1874, at the age of twenty-one, he took the diploma of the Society of Apothecaries. The following year he passed the examination to become a member of the Royal College of Surgeons. He then undertook a term of duty as a house surgeon at the London Hospital to build on his experience before accepting an offer from his elder brother, who was now honorary surgeon to the Royal National Hospital for Scrofula at Margate, down in Kent. At that hospital, though for only a few months, Frederick Treves became the resident medical officer. Even in this short time he managed to apply himself to an intensive study of scrofula, then still a disease of unknown origin.

By 1877 he felt the time had arrived for him to try his hand at general practice. It was a difficult period in which to start such a career, capital being necessary either to buy a share in a practice or simply to support a young doctor as he built up a practice of his own. There were also many young doctors competing for the patronage of the wealthy patients who made such a career possible and profitable. At this point Treves married Anne Elizabeth Mason, the youngest daughter of a Dorchester merchant. It is known that she brought some private money to their marriage, so it was probably this which enabled the young couple to set up home in the small town of Wirksworth, Derbyshire. Here Treves bought his way into a partnership in an isolated community, set in one of the beautiful Derbyshire vales. The practice extended for many miles to take in neighbouring farms and villages. It looked as though a dream had been realized.

In the event, the idyll did not last long. His strong personality and the impression of confidence which he conveyed to the patients precipitated jealousies among his senior partners. Within a year he was back near London, attempting to set up in general practice in the suburb of Sydenham. The chance of becoming surgical registrar at the London Hospital when the position fell vacant in 1878 was, in the circumstances, too good to miss. The relatively humble post was literally to provide the springboard for his whole future career.

The rungs of the ladder which Treves now mounted were placed as follows. First, in 1879, he became assistant surgeon to the London Hospital, and shortly afterwards also an assistant at the Royal London Ophthalmic

Hospital. This led to his being made lecturer and demonstrator in anatomy to the London Hospital Medical School, a position which he used to pioneer research in the whole new range of abdominal operations which anaesthesia and new antiseptic techniques were making possible. He wrote up his research notes from his work on scrofula, and these provided him with the material for his first book, *Scrofula and Its Gland Diseases* (1882).

Treves was now able to live up to the aspiration of owning a home in Bloomsbury, where he occupied 18 Gordon Square with his wife and two baby daughters. Other honours and publications followed, and he found that he could only get through all his commitments by observing a stringent self-discipline, rising as early as five or six each morning to write, study or catch up on correspondence before proceeding to his main duties of lecturing and operating throughout the day in the Medical School. The surgeon's task was heavy and exacting. One house governor of the London Hospital could recall how Treves's operating coat became so stiff with congealed blood that it stood upright without visible means of support when placed on the floor.

Already Treves had developed that combination of brusque directness with glimpsed moments of genuine if bluff human kindness which is associated in the public mind with eminent physicians. He became immensely popular with many of his students, to whom he preached a message of self-reliance: that they should rely on their judgement, make a firm decision and act on it without havering. The student who said to him one day about a case, 'It might be a fracture, sir, or it might be only sprained,' was sharply told: 'The patient is not interested to know it might be measles or it might be toothache. The patient wants to know what is the matter, and it is your business to tell him or he will go to a quack who will tell him at once.'

Despite his many professional duties, he still found time to speak for the Temperance Society on 'Alcohol: a Poison'; and to become chairman of the medical section of the Mission to Seamen. Then, with the year 1884, he was elected to the position of full consulting surgeon to the London Hospital.

Another change of life-style was necessary. He must build up a private consulting practice to bring him fees to make up for the fact that this was not a salaried post, though he would continue to receive fees for his teaching and, of course, royalties from his published writings. Promptly he moved his family from Bloomsbury to 6 Wimpole Street, where he was able to have consulting rooms in the heart of the Harley Street area.

It was a period of industrial depression, when few working-class families had as much to live on as £1 10s (£1.50) a week. Yet, Treves knew, at least one of his colleagues at the hospital, Sir Andrew Clark, was earning over £12,000 a year. 'Considering the number of patients who can comfortably be seen between nine and two o'clock and the number of visits that can be managed between two and seven,' Sir Andrew once wistfully remarked, 'I see no hope of improving that figure.' On the other hand, income tax had just been reduced from 8d. to 7d. in the pound.

The world, in a very real sense, was on the verge of opening up as Treves's oyster. And this was precisely the stage which his life had reached on the day when young Dr Tuckett told him about the strange Elephant Man in the freakshow across the road from the London Hospital, and was persuasive enough to make him decide to go and see for himself.

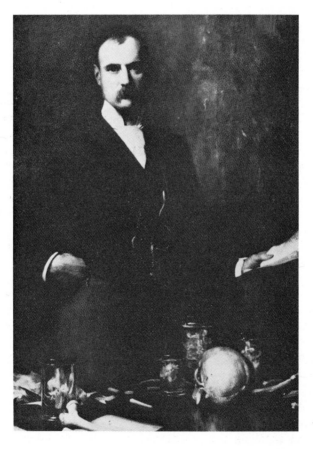

Plate 11. Sir Frederick Treves in the portrait by Luke Fildes which hangs in the Medical College of the London Hospital

CHAPTER 3

A Living Specimen

Eventually they stood facing each other, in Treves's room in the Anatomical Department of the Medical School.

We can only guess at what the freak from the exhibition shop may have made of Frederick Treves, this tall young surgeon, broad-shouldered and athletic in build, intensely observant and self-assured, possessing indeed a master's sailing certificate for his recreational yachting activities on the Dorset coast; a man who had already witnessed in his professional life most of the varieties of disease and physical distortion that can be induced by environment, behaviour or genetic misfortune in the slums of the world's greatest metropolis, but who had never come across anything quite like the Elephant Man before.

By contrast, we do know what Frederick Treves made of Joseph Merrick, as he measured him up and stripped him finally naked to the point where he was fully revealed as the most bizarre spectacle. Yet, of the man himself, he says little. 'He was shy, confused, not a little frightened and evidently much cowed. Moreover, his speech was unintelligible . . . I supposed that Merrick was imbecile and had been imbecile from birth.' The emphasis of the examination was on the physical aspects: to pass a tape measure round the head and limbs, finger the skin, assess the movement of the joints, hold back the shapeless blubber of the lips with a spatula to examine the inside of the mouth. There were massive abnormalities of the skin and flesh as well as some obvious and extraordinary distortions in bone structure. Meticulously, Treves charted every feature, recorded every peculiarity that he could discover on the appalling map of Merrick's body, but seemed to have hardly begun to draw any nearer to extracting a certainty of explanation from this chaotic anatomical wilderness.

The proportions were grotesque: a measurement of 36 inches was recorded for the head's circumference, another of 12 inches for that of the right wrist and one of 5 inches for the most swollen finger of the right hand. Yet Merrick was a short man, scarcely more than 5 feet 2 inches in height. In the skin Treves felt he could recognize two distinct abnormalities. First, there was an abnormality of the soft, subcutaneous tissue which lies immediately beneath the skin. It seemed in places to have greatly increased in quantity so that in these regions the skin was raised up above the surrounding tissue. Where this happened, the skin was very loose upon the body so that it could be made to slide about quite easily, or be grasped and drawn away from the deeper tissue in folds.

In three areas these changes were so marked that the weight of the skin drew the tissues down into pendulous folds that virtually hung like curtains of flesh from the body. One of these folds, about six inches square, hung in front of the right armpit, taking its root from the surface of the right breast and shoulder. A similar but less conspicuous fold hung down behind the armpit. It was in the buttocks, however, that the process was most marked, for here the skin flap was so thick and extensive that at first sight it looked as though the buttocks themselves descended in a great fold that reached almost to the level of the mid-thigh. So heavy and awkward was this fold of flesh that it tended to interfere with the functioning of the bowel and the action of defecation.

The second abnormality that Treves recognized in the skin was the presence of numerous warty growths or papillomata. These varied in size from being small, pimple-like roughenings of the skin to huge, cauliflower-textured masses. Their size and number varied between different areas of the body. In fact, the skin of the left arm was free from blemish, and parts of the face, and the eyelids and ears, seemed unaffected; the penis and scrotum were perfectly normal. Over the chest and abdomen the warts were small and sparse, but over the back of the head, and from between the shoulder blades down to the lower back and buttocks, they spread out as exuberant growths of dusky, purplish skin, deeply cleft and fissured. From the largest of these warty growths there rose the exceedingly foul odour which Treves first noticed in the shop where Merrick was exhibited.

If the skin changes made Joseph hideous, however, it was the skeletal changes which made him misshapen; but again, not all of the body was affected. Metamorphoses in the bones seemed to be limited to the skull, the bones of the right arm and hand and those of each leg below the knee.

The skull was enormous. It was completely irregular in shape, its surface being covered by huge rounded bosses of bone, some of them larger than

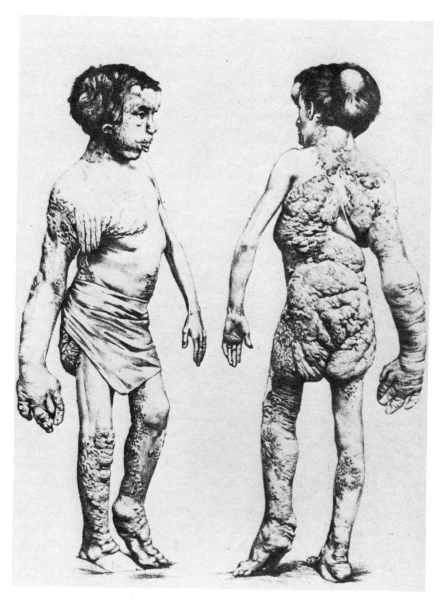

Plate 12. The earliest engravings, showing Joseph Merrick in 1884, from Treves's case presentation to the Pathological Society of London, as reproduced in the *Transactions* for 1885

tangerines. The most conspicuous bony lump stood out on the brow, but there were others to the side and back of the head. The whole left side of the head actually seemed to bulge out immediately above the ear, so that the ear was itself folded downwards almost at right angles to the head. It was extremely difficult, however, to trace the complete surface of the skull with any precision, for over most of the scalp the skin had produced its cauliflower-like masses and folds of loose skin in abundance.

The bones of the face were similarly distorted. The forehead was unduly large, uneven and rather protuberant, so that the eyes appeared small and set deeply back in the head. The bones of the right cheek were also much enlarged, so that the cheek was hard and prominent. The swelling had here pushed the hard palate forward and down, and forced the nose and mouth somewhat over to the left. When the mouth was open, it was possible to see a scar where a piece of tissue had evidently been removed at some time by an operation; the lower jaw seemed quite normal.

The right arm was greatly inflated, being two or three times the size of its fellow. Treves gained the impression that every bone in the limb, apart from the shoulder blade and collar bone, was uniformly enlarged, but there were none of those knobbly swellings upon the bones which were so prominent in the skull. The fantastic distortions of the bones had almost crippled the arm, for when Treves tried to manipulate it he found that while it could be moved fairly freely at the shoulder and elbow, the wrist and fingers were so stiff as to make the hand almost useless. Merrick could not, for example, turn his hand over and back again. The hand meanwhile was weirdly deformed, its huge misshapen fingers crowding one another into deformity and even partial dislocation of the joints. Strangely enough, though, the finger nails on the hand were perfect. As if in deliberate contrast, the left arm was completely unaffected, having a delicacy and neatness of proportion that made Treves think of the arm of a young girl.

Both the feet were distorted in a manner similar to the right arm, the bones being uniformly enlarged and the toes malformed and enormous. Merrick's posture illustrated the presence of the old disease of his left hip that Treves had already diagnosed, for he stood with his left leg held stiffly forward and away from the body. Apart from the tell-tale sign of a former hip disease and the various changes to the skin and bones, however, Treves could find little else that seemed to be amiss. The irony was that the Elephant Man apparently enjoyed good health in all other respects, suffering from no serious illness apart from his mysterious condition and even possessing an appreciable muscular strength.

As the examination and interview proceeded, so Treves became more accustomed to the Elephant Man's distorted and fluting voice and was able to add a little to his background knowledge of the man. The operation to the upper jaw, he gathered, had been carried out a year or two before in Leicester Infirmary. A developing tumour of the connective tissue in this area apparently grew to the point where it projected so far beyond the mouth that Merrick could no longer close his lips or masticate or move his jaw effectively. The surgeons at Leicester had therefore given him advice that it should be cut away.

Treves tried to discover whether there was any evidence for similar deformities occurring in Merrick's family, but there had apparently been none. It seems that Merrick stated he had neither brother nor sister, though, as will be seen shortly, the information was inaccurate. The head, right arm and feet had been badly deformed for as long as Merrick could remember, but when he was a child his skin was no more than roughened, loose and rather thick. The story of the profound shock suffered by his mother when bowled over by a circus elephant was again offered as a helpful clue.

In writing his essay on 'The Elephant Man', Treves conveys the impression that he returned Merrick to the care of the showman at the end of the day, once he had completed his examination, and that that was the last he saw of him during the present stage of the story. Again this is a simplification of events for the sake of narrative conciseness. He must, in fact, have remained in touch with Joseph Merrick and Tom Norman over the course of at least several days. Some time during this period, if not during the initial clinical interview, he must have arranged for the first photographs to be taken. He also persuaded Mr Norman (no doubt for an appropriate consideration) to allow his charge to be brought as a case for discussion and diagnosis before the eminent members of a learned medical society, the Pathological Society of London.

Perhaps at this point there was awakened in poor Joseph Merrick's heart, if not the wild hope of a cure, at least the chance of a wise and informed explanation or the assurance that something could be done to halt the advance of his disease. To have allowed himself to be exhibited before a group of medical mandarins might, in any case, have been no worse a prospect than exposing himself to the ill-informed curiosity of the majority of freakshow patrons.

Meetings of the Pathological Society of London were held on alternate Tuesday evenings at 8.30, at the headquarters of the society at 53 Berners Street, in Bloomsbury. Advance notice of meetings was always given in the *British Medical Journal*, together with a list of cases to be presented; it was also usual for a summary of any meeting to appear in the journal's following issue.

The *British Medical Journal* for 29 November 1884 was already in the press with its notice of the next meeting and the seven items listed for exhibition. Mr Frederick Treves was down simply to display two cases of tumour of the palate. He must have moved quickly, uncertain over how long he could remain effectively in touch with a case as peripatetic as a travelling freakshow exhibit. He therefore sought and gained permission to display Joseph as an additional item at the next meeting, on Tuesday, 2 December.

The Pathological Society of London was a highly respected institution. It had already been in existence for thirty-eight years, and it flourished right through to 1932, when it voluntarily disbanded so that it might be reconstituted as the Pathological Section of the present Royal Society of Medicine. It drew members not only from among London pathologists, surgeons and physicians, but also from doctors working in many of the leading provincial medical centres. A number of the society's members were not only eminent in the field of medicine, but were also associated with the realms of biology and the related sciences.

At all events, on 2 December Joseph Merrick was duly conveyed during the evening from Whitechapel to Bloomsbury. It must have surprised him somewhat to find himself the only living exhibit presented, or, for that matter, the only complete exhibit there. All other displays consisted merely of organs or sections of tissue removed from patients during an operation or at a post mortem.

Joseph's appearance as he entered the room certainly caused a stir among the society's members. The most astonished of them all was John Bland-Sutton, the young assistant surgeon from the Middlesex Hospital who chanced on the Elephant Man's freakshow before Treves.

> My surprise was great [he wrote] a fortnight later to find this man exhibited by Treves at the Pathological Society of London. He not only submitted Merrick for examination by members of the Society, but published a detailed and illustrated account of this unfortunate man in the *Transactions* for 1885.

Is there just a hint in this comment that Bland-Sutton felt Treves was being a little flamboyant in his choice of a case; that it lay perhaps on the borderline of medical discretion to have done so; that there was maybe even a touch of the showman's instincts in the action?

The fact remains that while the Elephant Man may have been seen in his freakshow by other gifted medical personalities, it was Treves who took the step of deciding that here was a case which demanded explanation. Even so, apart from the first murmurs of surprise, there seems to have been little response from members of the Pathological Society. No one came forward with any constructive suggestion, and the problem of diagnosis was carried no further. The digest of the meeting which appeared in the *British Medical Journal* for the following week simply stated:

> *Congenital Deformity* – MR TREVES showed a man who presented an extraordinary appearance, owing to a series of deformities: some congenital exostoses of the skull; extensive papillomatous growths and large pendulous masses in connection with the skin; great enlargement of the right upper limb, involving all the bones. From the massive distortion of the head, and the extensive areas covered by papillomatous growth, the patient had been called 'the elephant-man'.

The correspondent for the *Lancet* clearly shared Bland-Sutton's reservations about the propriety of demonstrating such a sensational case before the society. In a very lengthy account of the meeting which the journal published, there is no mention whatsoever of Joseph's presence.

It seemed that Treves was fated to be left with his original, vague diagnosis of a congenital deformity, and that Joseph, none the wiser for his brief sojourn among higher medical authorities, must return to the care of Mr Tom Norman and the relentless round of earning his living on the freakshow circuits. For most doctors, that would have been the end of their attempts to solve such a puzzle; but Frederick Treves was nothing if not determined.

Four months later he tried again. It was just possible that, by putting the case forward one more time, after giving adequate notice in the medical journals, some doctor or specialist with knowledge of this strange condition might be encouraged to attend the meeting; or, alternatively, that the lapse of time might have allowed some of those who had seen Joseph Merrick to have considered the problem at leisure.

By now Treves knew nothing of the whereabouts of Merrick and Tom Norman, but he had the photographs and he had the data and clinical findings from his first examination. These he was able to present to the meeting of the Pathological Society of London which was held on Tuesday, 17 March 1885. And on this occasion his endeavours attracted a response, for among those gathered for the meeting was Dr Henry Radcliffe Crocker.

Radcliffe Crocker was then just forty years old, a physician from University College Hospital, London, who had specialized in diseases of the skin, having as a student come under the influence of the late Dr Tilbury Fox, a dermatologist who had attempted to reduce the problems of dermatology to a semblance of scientific order. Tilbury Fox soon infected the younger doctor with enthusiasm for his speciality, and within a few years Radcliffe Crocker was coming to be recognized among the world's leading authorities on skin diseases.

After listening to Treves's presentation of the Elephant Man's case in silence, Dr Radcliffe Crocker rose to make his own observations. His dissertation was quietly brilliant. Surely, he suggested, this was no new or undescribed disease. It seemed a case that must surely be classified as belonging to that rare group of disorders known as *dermatolysis* (a loosened or pendulous condition of the skin) and *pachydermatocoele* (a condition where tumours arise from an overgrowth of skin). Both these skin disorders, though excessively rare, had been known for some years.

It was Dr Radcliffe Crocker's opinion that these two forms of skin disorder were in some way related, that an association was already recognized between them by the medical profession; for, on one or two other occasions, as in Treves's case, they had been found to coexist in the same patient. He felt that the particular interest in the example of the Elephant Man lay in the fact that he presented a third feature: a deformity of the bones. The combination of the skin conditions with bone changes was something that, so far as he knew, had never before been described.

Having linked up three pieces in the bizarre medical jigsaw, Radcliffe Crocker, before he sat down, rounded off his remarks with an inspired suggestion. He reminded the meeting of a case presented before the society by his old mentor, Dr Tilbury Fox, where a patient with the symptoms of a looseness of the skin had developed these after an injury and a resulting abscess which needed to be lanced. It was found that the parts of the body affected were those supplied by the nerves damaged by the injury and the subsequent abscess. Could it not therefore be that changes in the nervous system had governed the bodily distribution of the disease in the Elephant Man?

It was still vague enough, and it still left many questions unanswered, but with the hindsight of almost a century it is possible to say that it was a better explanation than Treves had any right to expect. The Pathological Society of London and Dr Radcliffe Crocker had provided as accurate an answer as it would have been possible to give anywhere in the world in the state of medical knowledge as it existed in 1885.

What, in the meantime, of Joseph Merrick and Mr Norman? The tide of rational decency was by now running heavily against their interconnected interests. Even in the East End of London, a new sensitivity in public opinion was leading to demands for official action to be taken to shut down exhibitions which were found by a growing number of citizens to be offensive. It was all part of a long and, it has to be said, civilizing process. The 'taste for Monsters' which, Henry Morley wrote, 'became a disease' during the heyday of Bartholomew Fair, was one 'of which the nation has in our own day [the 1850s] recovered with a wonderful rapidity'. During Queen Anne's reign, at the house next to the Greyhound Inn during Bartholomew Fair, there was an exhibition of a hydrocephalic child: 'but Thirty weeks old, with a prodigious big head, being above a yard about, and hath been shown to several Persons of Quality'. There can be few societies today in which an attempt to put on such an exhibition would be greeted with anything but outrage.

There have always been, however, two sides to the question whenever righteous indignation has succeeded in imposing its general will. In his book *The Travelling People*, Duncan Dallas records the lamentation of one present-day fairground showman who was having much difficulty in finding an adequate supply of human freaks. He blamed it on the Welfare State in Britain: '. . . you never hear anything about these people. They seem to be smothered. They seem to be kept out of the way in the background.'

The implication is that freaks still exist in plenty, but that society would prefer not to have the discomfort of knowing about them. The old showmen, including Tom Norman, were naturally at one in claiming that their freaks were better off out in the world, among people and earning a living, than shut away in an institution or an isolated home from which they could never venture forth, dependent on charity or welfare. So where should the line be drawn between the object of legitimate curiosity and the offence to public decency?

There was no question in the minds of the London police but that Joseph Merrick came well within the latter category. They had therefore stepped in to close down the show in the Whitechapel Road as they would, only three years later on the same site, close down the waxworks exhibition on the theme of the Jack the Ripper murders. Joseph and Mr Norman had retreated back along the road out of the metropolis and disappeared somewhere in the provincial background, and Frederick Treves had no reason to think that he might ever have dealings with either of them again.

Meanwhile there were his notes and data as well as the photographs, and there was one further task which he intended to undertake. This was to prepare his account of the case for publication in the *Transactions of the Pathological Society of London*. Copies of the photographs were sent to Messrs F. Huth, Lithographers, of Edinburgh, and eventually the finished plates, together with Treves's description, were published in the *Transactions* for 1885 under the heading, 'A Case of Congenital Deformity'.

Thus Treves had made a permanent record of the case to be bequeathed to medical posterity and taken up by any expert who might in the future feel drawn to unravelling its mysteries. By now he was busily engaged in delivering the Hunterian Lectures on Anatomy to the Royal College of Surgeons, and if he thought further of the Elephant Man it was to hope that his impression of him as a retarded individual was an accurate one.

The fact that his face was incapable of expression, that his speech was a mere spluttering and his attitude that of one whose mind was void of all emotions and concerns gave grounds for this belief. The conviction was no doubt encouraged by the hope that his intellect was the blank I imagined it to be.

The possibility that Joseph Merrick could after all have any realization of the dilemma of his life would, Treves felt, be unthinkable.

CHAPTER 4

A Parade of Elephants
and Early Griefs

What, then, is known or can be discovered of the origins of Joseph Merrick?

His birth certificate gives the information that he was born Joseph Carey Merrick on 5 August 1862 at 50 Lee Street, Leicester; that his father was Joseph Rockley Merrick, warehouseman, and his mother Mary Jane Merrick, née Potterton. As the date of their marriage in the parish church of Thurmaston was 29 December 1861, it is fair to assume that Mary Jane was already pregnant by the time she went to the altar. She was twenty-six years old when she gave birth to Joseph, and his memory of her was, as we shall see, one of the most important elements in his life.

An anonymous article on the Elephant Man which appeared in the *Illustrated Leicester Chronicle* on 27 December 1930, which was clearly based on a knowledge of the Merrick family circumstances (though its source is now untraceable), stated that Mary Jane was herself a cripple. She was born in the small village of Evington on the outskirts of Leicester, the eldest child in a family of six. Her parents, William and Elizabeth Potterton, were ordinary country people. Indeed, her father, a farm labourer, could not write his own name, but the Pottertons did well by their children, allowing them to attend school until they received at least a basic education.

When Mary was about seven years old, her family moved from Evington to settle in the village of Thurmaston, a few miles to the north of Leicester. From there, at the age of twelve, she left home to become a servant to a family which lived in Leicester itself.

For the next thirteen years she remained in service, enduring a life that must have been distinctive only for its long hours and attic bedrooms, the endless carrying of hot-water jugs and coal buckets, incessant scrubbing and blackleading and the inevitable rules about 'no followers'.

Columns :—	1	2	3	4	5
No.	When and where born	Name, if any	Sex	Name, and surname of father	Name, surname, and m surname of mothe
395	Fifth August 1862 50 Lee Street	Joseph Carey	Boy	Joseph Rockley Merrick	Mary Jane Merrick former Potter

Plate 13. The birth entry for Joseph Carey Merrick, reproduced from the local register

Then, in 1861, when she was twenty-five years old, she met Joseph Rockley Merrick. He worked as the driver of a brougham, a four-wheeled cab, and was a little more than a year younger than Mary. His family had also been agricultural labourers, at Bulcote, near Nottingham, but they forsook the land to migrate to Leicester before Joseph Rockley was born. His father, Barnabus Merrick, was now employed in the hosiery trade as a bobbin-maker. After their marriage, the young Merricks set up their first home together at 50 Lee Street, in a small house that lay in one of the crowded streets behind Humberstonegate and which was only a few yards from the house of Joseph's parents.

The city of Leicester was expanding rapidly on the basis of the industrial-ization of its traditional crafts of hosiery and knitwear, to which were added boot and shoe manufacture. Fresh mazes of narrow streets and dingy back-to-back housing would spring up with regularity in each succeeding year. From the north side of Humberstonegate, a long, narrow street called Wharf Street ran down at right angles to reach the new public wharf on the canal. The land to each side of Wharf Street was low-lying and even marshy, but by the 1860s the gardens and nurseries still charted on the maps of 1828 had disappeared beneath a confusion of backstreets. Lee Street was one of these: a side-turning off Wharf Street.

From its moment of construction Lee Street could be justly defined as a slum. The houses were small and they lacked running water. Sanitation was a constant problem, for the sewers were inadequate and many houses pos-

6	7	8	9	10*
Occupation of father	Signature, description, and residence of informant	When registered	Signature of registrar	Name entered after registration
warehouseman	*M 2 Merrick* *Mother* *60 Lee Street* *Leicester.*	*Twentysixth* *August* *1862*	*Robert* *Warburton* *Registrar*	*001*

sessed only cesspits. The removal of refuse was left to private scavengers, who were both ineffective and irregular. Worst of all, however, were the floods. Once a year the River Soar and the canal could be expected to rise and fill the streets to a depth of two or three feet, the water having forced its way back up through the sewers, bringing with it sewage and garbage. It was both insanitary and lethal. Over many years Leicester was to suffer a death-rate which annually removed between twenty-six and thirty in every thousand of its population; and, as always, the death-rate was highest among infants and children. Those Victorian mothers had little hope of being spared the helpless agony of watching at least one of their children sicken and die.

Shortly after his marriage, Joseph Rockley Merrick changed his job. He gave up his employment as a brougham driver and went to work in one of the many cotton factories. The work would have been monotonous and the hours long, the usual shift lasting from 8 a.m. to 7 p.m. in winter and from 6 a.m. to 5.30 p.m. in summer, with half an hour for breakfast and dinner. Many firms already allowed Saturday afternoons as a half-day, but there were no statutory bank holidays and even Boxing Day was regarded as a normal day of work. Wages varied somewhat, but a man working two knitting frames could earn as much as 12s. (60p) or 15s. (75p) a week, a woman 9s. (45p) and even a child might bring home 2s. (10p) or 3s. (15p). Joseph Rockley Merrick was somewhat more fortunate, however, for he managed to obtain a job in the warehouse where the wages were slightly higher than those paid to the actual operatives, the men and women who worked in the warehouse generally being regarded as a better class of employee.

In Leicester, Mary came under the influence of the Baptist ministry, which was particularly strong in the town, and for a period in her life she was a teacher in one of the three Baptist Sunday schools in the city, though which one is uncertain. Education in Leicester, as in many of the other new and growing industrial centres, presented a considerable problem in the 1860s. Children of seven and eight years old were still being employed by the cotton factories, by the boot manufacturers and in the brickyards. There were no free schools prior to the Education Act of 1870, and parents could often not afford to pay even the small fees charged by the various day schools, apart from their unwillingness to sacrifice the wages of their earning children. In fact, only a third of the children in Leicester received a full-time education, and many of these attended for such short periods that they can have gained little benefit.

For the rest of the children there were the Sunday schools, usually run by the Nonconformist churches. The purpose of them was to teach not only religious instruction, but also the rudiments of reading, writing and arithmetic. While we do not know which Baptist Sunday school employed Mary's services, the activities of the Friar Lane Baptist Sunday School give an indication that the régime was a stern business, whatever benevolent motivation the Nonconformist conscience must have had in working for the betterment of working-class children.

The Sunday schools were often surprisingly large establishments, the one at Friar Lane having as many as 350 pupils and 45 teachers. Admission was a matter of application and interview, and truancy led to expulsion, for discipline was strict. At the beginning of the nineteenth century this school had even possessed a pair of stocks for the correction of the unruly. Successful scholars could, however, look forward to prize day and receiving certificates of proficiency; and there was always the annual Sunday school outing.

The relentlessly harsh work routine for the populace of the industrial centres of the nineteenth century naturally created, by reaction, an appetite for diversion and cheap entertainment during the few hours which people could call their own. The 1860s were the first great period of growth for the institution of the British music hall throughout the provinces, though many of the new halls were still attached as incidental attractions to existing inns and taverns. There were meanwhile the more traditional diversions whose origins went far back into antiquity: the charter fairs and visiting circuses and menageries, the latter, of course, featuring elephants among their attractions. And the mention of elephants at once creates an echo in the mind: the carefully tended story which Joseph Merrick put forward to account for his condition, that his mother had been knocked down by an elephant during the time she was pregnant with him.

The *Leicester Journal* for 9 May 1862 contained the following announcement:

Notice is hereby given that the next Leicester MAY FAIR will be held on Monday, the 12th day of May next for the sale of horses, beasts and sheep, and on Tuesday, the 13th and following days for the sale of cheese. By order, Saul Stone, Town Clerk. N.B. No cheese wagon will be allowed to enter the Market Place except from Hotel Street.

The following day the *Leicester Chronicle* dutifully repeated the notice.

There were fairs in Leicester from the thirteenth century. The dates of the fairs, and the festivals which they celebrated, had varied over the years, but gradually they all coalesced into the two great annual fairs of the city. The first was held early in the May of each year, at the time of the 'Invention of the Cross'; the second in early October at Michaelmas. Before their discontinuation in 1902, they were among the truly great charter fairs of Britain. People came pouring into the city from the neighbouring villages and towns to buy and sell in the markets, hire employees and domestic staff and watch the quality and prices of cattle and horses. They replenished farmhouse stocks for another six months, exchanged domestic news with neighbours, bought new clothes and marvelled at the new fashions, pushed their way between the street stalls and ended up revelling in the tomfooleries of the Pleasure Fair.

For the citizens of Leicester, the fairs were a mixed blessing as the streets and thoroughfares became blocked by stalls and surging crowds. Cotton spinners hurrying in the early morning to the small factories and mills would find their way blocked by the cattle being driven through to the Cattle Market in the city centre. For two days the streets became treacherous and foul. As Dr John Barclay of Leicester remarked in a lecture which he delivered in 1864:

That the cattle market is a terrible nuisance no one will, I think, deny. I am sure that no one will say a word in support of it who have to barricade their doors against the filthy accumulations that make the streets look and smell like a cowshed for a couple of days. In my own part of the town we are quite blockaded ...

No sooner were the cattle sales over than the poultry came into town the next day, noisy and living in the backs of a hundred carts. Then there would be comparative peace and cleanliness as the cheese fair took over. From every farm and dairy the great cheeses were brought, laid on fresh straw in the bottoms of carts. From end to end of the town the carts, their horses unharnessed, stood backed against the kerbs, tailboards lowered to display their cheeses to passers-by. Shopkeepers and housewives alike would move along the line, tasting samples before buying. The best cheeses went quickly to the large grocers; only the worst cheeses would still be left when the gas lamps were lit at early dusk.

In the meantime, as the trading fairs proceeded, the Humberstonegate, as one of the wider thoroughfares of the town, was set aside for the great pleasure fair. Stalls and booths were ranged down either side of the street,

Plate 14. The scene in Humberstonegate, Leicester, during the May fair, photographed at the turn of the century

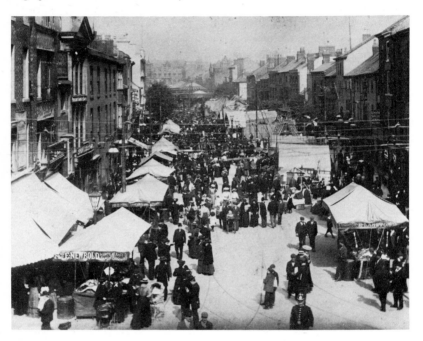

and where the road widened into its broadest part, there were swings and merry-go-rounds; theatrical booths and marionettes; freakshows, sword swallowers and jugglers; stands for the sale of sweets, pastries and patent medicines.

Mrs I.C. Ellis, in her collection of reminiscences, *Nineteenth Century Leicester*, remembered it thus:

> The fair in Humberstonegate was a glimpse of paradise. It was a never forgotten joy to go on the roundabouts though we never ventured

on the swings. The wild beast show roared and smelt like nothing else on earth, but the daintiest, loveliest thing was the marionette show. We were taken down the bazaars – and very nice the stalls were – a long row of tents with wares all on one side ... There were booths with dancers in tights disporting themselves on a platform – these our father or other conductor avoided, but the marionettes we were allowed to see ... We went to front seats (2d. by the side door, 1d. if you went in at the front, in view of all the fair). When we had all been paid for and were sitting as we thought in seclusion, the proprietor opened the front of this tent and displayed his respectable audience, and shouted again, 'Twopence in at the side door, one penny in at the front.'

In its report of the 1862 pleasure fair, the *Leicester Journal* succeeded enthusiastically in putting over the excited flavour:

> Giants, descendants in direct line from the Anakims of old; india-rubber men; or acrobats; wonders of every description in animated nature, and astonishing novelties in art, are presented. A picture of a monstrous pig, exhibited outside one booth, is said to have its perfect living counterpart weighing several tons within. At another booth resides a cow, whose hind quarters are adorned with an extra leg, which the proprietor informs us, is intended expressly for scratching her nose.

The *Leicester Chronicle*, as it took up the theme, was altogether more concerned to avoid being carried away.

> Not withstanding the heavy showers of rain and the somewhat limited attractions ... it has been visited by a large number of the country folk during the week ... There was a new circus, Croueste's, displaying to the admiring gaze of the juveniles a number of coloured vignettes, representing equestrians in all sorts of impossible attitudes; and a dilapidated theatrical booth, with actors and actresses, whose dresses were in admirable keeping with the woe-begone appearance of the building. A giant pig, a threelegged cow, some dirty looking and rickety swingboats, really superior roundabouts, stalls for nick-nacks, and rifle galleries – made up a somewhat motley gathering of the peripatetic tradesfolk.

Yet this paragraph also contains what is, from the point of view of the present account, one plum of information: 'The principal feature has been, of course, Wombwell's Menagerie ...' The wild-beast show could hardly manage to fail. Permanent collections of animals were still extremely rare, so the only opportunity which most people had of seeing zoological specimens from exotic parts was offered by the travelling menageries. There were in the country several different companies on the road each year, including Atkins's and Sedgwick's, but perhaps the most famous in the annals of fairground history was Wombwell's Royal Menagerie.

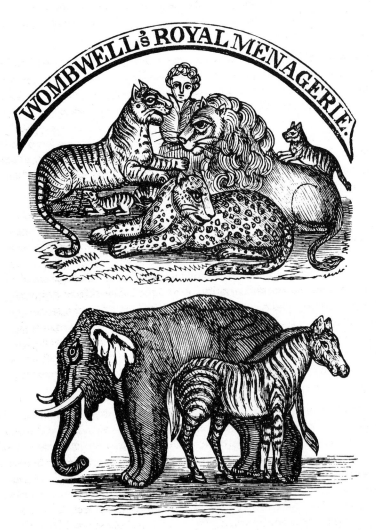

Plate 15. Design from a broadsheet advertising Wombwell's Royal Menagerie (reproduced from Morley's *Memoirs of Bartholomew Fair*, 1880)

It was founded in 1807 by George Wombwell, of whom William Hone spoke ill when he encountered him at Bartholomew Fair in 1825:

> ... he ... exhibited himself, to my judgment of him, with an understanding and feelings perverted by avarice. He is undersized in mind as well as in form, 'a weazen, sharp-faced man', with a skin reddened by more than natural spirits, and he speaks in a voice and language that accord with his feelings and propensities.

Hone also held against Wombwell a disgraceful event a short while before at Warwick, where the publicity-hungry proprietor set up a gladiatorial combat in which his two lions, Nero and Wallace, were baited by dogs. Despite (or because of) such episodes, Wombwell's flourished, growing ultimately into three separate touring menageries and on five occasions receiving a royal command, thrice to appear before Queen Victoria herself.

Thomas Frost, author of *The Old Showmen and the Old London Fairs*, has left a memory from boyhood of the magic anticipation which Wombwell's aroused for him at Croydon Fair:

> I ... could never sufficiently admire the gorgeously uniformed bandsmen, whose brazen instruments brayed and blared from noon till night on the exterior platform, and the immense pictures, suspended from lofty poles, of elephants and giraffes, lions and tigers, zebras, boa constrictors, and whatever else was most wonderful in the brute creation, or most susceptible of brilliant colouring. The difference in scale to which the zoological rarities within were depicted on the canvas, as compared with the figures of the men that were represented, was a very characteristic feature of these pictorial displays. The boa constrictor was given the girth of an ox, and the white bear should have been as large as an elephant, judged by the size of the sailors who were attacking him among his native ice-bergs.

Curiously enough, so far as elephants went, they always figured largely in anecdotes of Wombwell's exploits. On one occasion he mistimed his tour and, says Thomas Frost, was still in Newcastle-upon-Tyne with no more than two weeks to go before the opening of Bartholomew Fair in London. The possibility of his reaching London in time with his procession of caged beasts along the roads of those days therefore looked remote in the extreme. At this point Wombwell gained wind of the fact that his arch-rival, Atkins, was promoting his menagerie at Bartholomew's as 'the only wild beast show in the fair'. Without hesitation Wombwell undertook an epic forced march to bring his caravanserai to London on the day the fair opened; but the effort took its toll of the elephant. The poor beast dropped dead on arrival. Atkins thereupon lost not a moment in declaiming that he had 'the only living elephant in the fair'; at which Wombwell counter-attacked with his slogan: 'The only dead elephant in the fair.' The tactic paid off, since, remarks Frost, a 'dead elephant was a greater rarity than a live one, and his show was crowded every day of the fair, while Atkins's was comparatively deserted'.

Plate 16. Bostock & Wombwell's Menagerie on the road, featuring the great procession of the beast wagons, traditional transport for a century

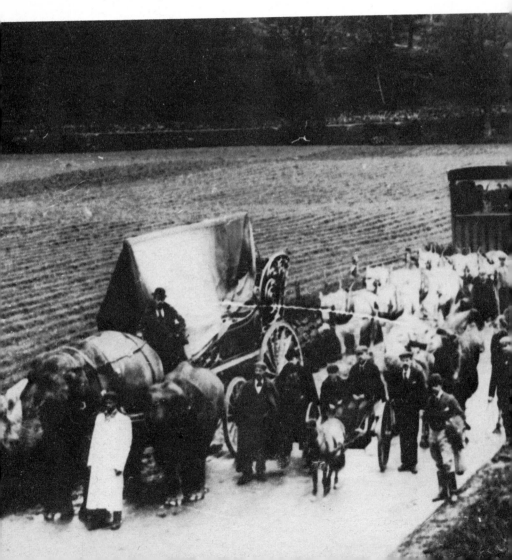

For the Bartholomew Fair of 1830, Wombwell's proudest boast was the Elephant of Siam, 'a theatrical performer', says Henry Morley, 'in the spectacle of the *Fire-fiend*, wherein it uncorked bottles and declaimed for the Rightful Prince. On each side of it he had in his show two miniature elephants, the "smallest ever seen in Europe".'

It was a Wombwell elephant, too, which once broke out of the fairground to take a leisurely stroll down Croydon High Street in the small hours of the morning, to the alarm and astonishment of the town constable. The animal stopped when it came to a confectioner's, butted in the shutters and window panes with its head and helped itself to cakes and dainties.

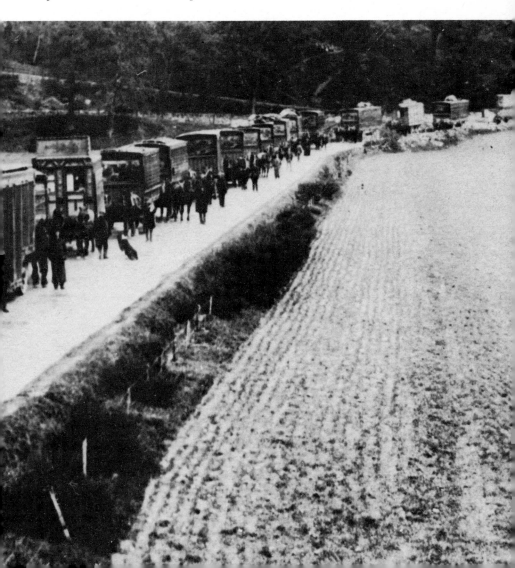

By 1862, when Wombwell's was travelling to Leicester for the May fair in Humberstonegate, old George had been dead a dozen years and the main company was under his widow's management. The routine leading up to the menagerie's arrival in town would, however, have been along the established pattern. First the advance agents arrived, to book the site, arrange water supplies and stabling, buy in corn and forage. The printers were commissioned to run off handbills, posters went up on walls and announcements were inserted on the front page of local newspapers whose inside columns carried news of the American Civil War.

Finally, on the first day of the fair, the town would find itself aroused at seven in the morning by the rattle and shaking of a column of heavy wagons in the streets. In the convoy were the accommodation caravans, the provision carts and seventeen or eighteen beast wagons, these last being cages on wheels, eight feet high and broad, and as much as eighteen feet long, their sides concealed by great shutters, their wheels iron-rimmed and noisy. The beast wagons came through the town with as many as four shire horses straining before each one, their hooves slipping and sparking on the cobbles; and marching between the wagons, sometimes hitched to one or other of the larger vehicles, there walked the elephants and camels.

Once in Humberstonegate, with a shouting and pushing of horses, the wagons were backed up to form a square, three sides formed by the wagons themselves, the fourth consisting of the high wooden façade which was the front of the show. On the outside, the façade was decorated with mock wooden pillars and painted panels on which enraged beasts fought in impossible jungles while men, magnificent in their bare-chested bravery, wrestled with ferocious lions. In the centre of the façade was the pay-box, perched high on a small platform, and when, at last, the square was complete, it was roofed over by canvas sheeting stretched from wagon to wagon. Finally, on the inside of the square, the yellow shutters of the beast wagons were lowered on their hinges to hide the wheels and reveal the occupants.

Up the steps and past the pay-box the customer could then duck through the curtains that screened the doorway to find himself at the head of the steps leading down into the covered square. Tethered here and there in small groups about the compound stood llamas and camels and other theoretically acquiescent creatures. In the cages about the square would be the wolves and leopards, bears, monkeys, zebras, small antelopes, parrots and pelicans. There might be a tiger, though this was a rather uncommon beast, the showmen finding them unpredictable and difficult to train. Two of the cages were for lions, in one of which the trainer would stand face to face with two or three of the great cats, making them pose, leap through hoops, lie down

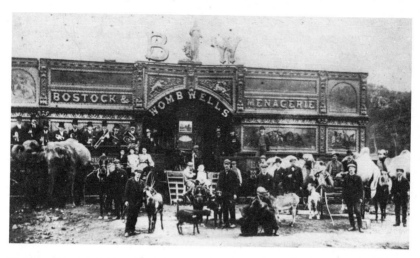

Plate 17. Bostock & Wombwell's menagerie set up for business in the 1900s with the band *in situ*

and stand up to command. But if the lions provided the thrills, it was the elephants which imparted a feeling of solid merit and spectacle. The local population would assess the status of any menagerie on the size and number of its elephants.

At midday on each day of the fair it was therefore customary to open the side gates of the menagerie so that the elephants might parade solemnly out, and move ponderously through the streets as an impressive walking advertisement. Their procession was one of the highlights of the pleasure fair, and the reporter from the *Leicester Journal* must have been speaking for many of his fellow citizens when he cheerfully summed it all up in the one phrase, that Wombwell's was here 'in all its glory'.

In the reports of the local press in Leicester for May 1862 there is, however, no mention of an unfortunate girl, crippled and pregnant, stumbling when forced by the crush of the crowd on to the roadway in front of the great feet of a parading elephant, falling down but scrambling clear, distressed and badly shaken. There is no reason why there should be a record of such an incident, nor any reason why anyone should have known about it afterwards, apart from the immediate bystanders. The fact remains that it has become an event so inextricably intertwined in the legend of the Elephant Man, an incident so often mentioned by those who were acquainted with Joseph Merrick, that it would be unreasonable to suppose it never occurred.

✳

Mary Jane Merrick gave birth to her first child three months after the Humberstonegate fair. He was christened Joseph after his father and for a second name his mother chose Carey, calling him after the leading Baptist preacher and missionary, William Carey (1761-1834), who had done so much to foster the Baptist ministry in Leicester and who not only founded the Baptist Missionary Society in London but was also one of its two first missionaries. Three weeks after her son was born, Mary herself attended at the Register Office to record the birth.

Mary and Joseph would at first have noticed no fault in their little boy. The anonymous but informative article which appeared in the *Illustrated Leicester Chronicle* in December 1930 stated that: '... the relatives declare that ... Merrick was born a perfect baby'. He must have seemed perfectly made, even delicately proportioned, and in spite of the dangers of the environment and an epidemic of smallpox which raged through Leicester the following year, Mary was spared the pain of losing him. He not only survived but would have seemed to flourish for a while.

Mary's joy, however, was destined to be short-lived. Her infant son was soon to begin to grow grotesquely deformed, each year of his life bringing with it an increased distortion and affliction. There is some confusion over the onset of Joseph's symptoms; available accounts vary greatly on the subject of when the first manifestations of his terrible disease became un-avoidably obvious. One writer, in the *British Medical Journal* of 19 April 1890, suggested that it was almost certain that the Elephant Man had been born with enlargement of the bones of the skull, right arm and feet. Yet Joseph himself wrote: 'It was not perceived much at birth, but began to develop itself when at the age of five years.' Once again it is the article in the *Illustrated Leicester Chronicle* which gives the only detailed account and the description which accords most closely with current understanding and experience of his strange disorder.

According to this article, it was when her baby was about twenty-one months old that Mary first became aware of something strange happening, of a firm swelling forming in his lower lip. During the next months, this would have increased in size, spreading up as a hard tumour into the right cheek, until the little child's upper lip was being pushed outwards by a mass of pink protruding flesh. Mary must then have been tormented by the gradual realization that there was something seriously abnormal about her boy and that the trouble showed no sign of passing. As he grew older, a bony lump appeared on the forehead, and this, too, increased perceptibly in size; his skin grew rather loose and rough in texture; even his bodily proportions were beginning to be marred by a peculiar enlargement of the right arm and both feet.

The question of Joseph Merrick's trouble in the light of informed, up-to-date medical opinion strictly speaking belongs later on in the book and is the subject of Chapter 10. For the moment it is sufficient to say that, in 1970, Dr Norman Fienman and Dr William Yakovac of the Children's Hospital of Philadelphia and the University of Pennsylvania published a study of this particular disorder as it can occur in childhood. They managed to investigate forty-six children who were suffering from the condition, but in no case did they see deformity of the skull or the bones of the limbs at birth. In twenty of their patients, however, they were able to diagnose the disease at birth, and in thirty-four children, or three-quarters of their total series, by the age of two. In forty children (86 per cent of their cases) the disease had betrayed its presence by the appearance of skin pigmentation or the development of tumours.

These observations were confirmed in 1972 by the late Dr Richard Brasfield and Dr Tapas Das Gupta of the Abraham Lincoln School of Medicine, Chicago, who published a survey of 110 cases. Their patients were drawn from every age group and included sixty children in whom the disease had occurred before the age of five. They had recognized abnormalities of the bones of the head and limbs in 47 per cent of their patients, but observed that the age at which these changes first appeared in a patient varied between six and thirty-five years. It would seem that, in mentioning the age of five, Joseph must himself have been referring to the onset of the deformities in the bones of his limbs and skull.

Among all the bizarre distortions which were afflicting the body of her child, the most terrible for Mary must surely have been the initial, extraordinary mass of flesh which continued to force its way from beneath the upper lip. It was eventually to protrude for several inches from his mouth in a grotesque snout weighing three or four ounces. To even the most unimaginative eye, the resemblance to an elephant's trunk must have been obvious. During all those early years, Mary's mind can only have gone ever more frequently back to her mishap with the elephant in Humberstonegate as she cast around helplessly to explain the inexplicable, to herself as much as to her relations and gossiping neighbours.

In the meantime, Joseph Rockley Merrick had moved house again, taking his family from Lee Street to their new home at 119 Upper Brunswick Street, Leicester. He had also changed jobs once more. The history of the hosiery industry in the first half of the nineteenth century is the story of its mechanization. Steam power changed the pattern of what was once a cottage industry, and by the 1860s one social observer in Leicester was able to count more than 250 factory chimneys on the city skyline. Joseph Rockley had found new employment as a stoker on a steam engine in one of the cotton factories.

Then, shortly after moving into her new home, Mary became pregnant for the second time, and on 8 January 1866 gave birth to her second son. This one she called William, after her own father, and added Arthur, a common name in the Merrick family. Any fears that she may have had that her second child would develop deformities similar to those crippling her firstborn proved groundless, for William Arthur's growth, it is said, remained free of abnormalities.

It was about this time that her elder son suffered a further misfortune when he fell heavily, damaging his left hip. After the injury the joint became diseased, and so he was left permanently lame by the accident. His appearance must already have been making it difficult for him to mix with other children; now it would have become impossible for him to join in their games since he could do little more than hobble. His mother doubtless tried to ensure that his life followed a pattern as close as possible to normal, for she sent him to school each day; but she must have known that the deformities were leaving their mark, that he was becoming a lonely, introspective child, isolated from his fellows and all the time increasingly dependent on the company of his mother.

On 28 September 1867, Mary gave birth to her third and last child. This time it was a daughter, who was duly christened Marion Eliza. Mary Jane Merrick's family was complete, and her husband gained further welcome promotion. Joseph Rockley Merrick could now classify himself as 'engine driver at the cotton factory'. He must, however, have been a restless and enterprising man since he soon began to make plans for a modest but independent commercial venture. In the *Leicester Trade Directory* for 1870 (prepared in 1869), his name appears as the proprietor of a haberdashery shop at 37 Russell Square, a small square which lay to the north end of Wharf Street. It was not that he had any intention of relinquishing his job at the factory, for this was to be one among many small 'back street' family enterprises planned to be run by a wife or relatives. As such it must have been at least moderately successful since it continued to gain mention in the *Leicester Trade Directories* right through until 1880. Meanwhile he moved his family once more, not to live in the house above the shop but to another house at 161 Birstall Street, a side street close to Russell Square.

The haberdashery shop was not in existence for long before serious troubles began to visit the family. In the period of preparation leading up to Christmas 1870, the Merricks' second child, little William Arthur, now nearly five years old, fell dangerously ill with scarlet fever. Within twenty-four hours his condition was surely desperate, and on 21 December he died. The following day Mary herself attended the Register Office to make notification of his death, and the death certificate bears mute witness to the devastation she felt at losing him. When she came to sign the document, Mary, the Sunday school teacher, the girl who had signed her name so confidently on her own marriage certificate and on each of the birth certificates of her children, could manage no more than a cross, identified by the registrar as 'the mark of Mary Jane Merrick, present at the death'.

While to lose a young child was then no uncommon experience, it would be presumptuous to take this as in any way lightening her pain. The one thing she would have had in which to bury her grief would have been her time-consuming round of responsibilities: a three-year-old daughter and a growing, crippled son, besides the management of the shop in Russell Square on her husband's behalf. It may be that her strength was at a low ebb by the spring of 1873, when she fell ill with bronchopneumonia. Her struggle with the disease did not last long, and in the early hours of Thursday, 19 May, she died. The day was her thirty-sixth birthday, and her son Joseph was then just three months short of reaching the age of eleven.

When he wrote 'The Elephant Man', Frederick Treves, on the basis of what he knew of Joseph Merrick and his past history, came to the conclusion that Joseph's memory of his mother as a beautiful woman who had loved him was a fantasy that he needed to sustain for psychological reasons, to counterbalance his own ugliness and the fact that 'since the day when he could toddle no one had been kind to him'. Mary Jane Merrick was thus dismissed as 'worthless and inhuman', a woman who 'basely deserted' her small son, abandoning him to the workhouse. In the perspective of the facts, this may now be seen as an unfortunate if unintended libel, and doubly unfortunate in that it posthumously compounded poor Mary Jane's personal tragedy.

CHAPTER 5

The Mercy of the Parish

To give Frederick Treves his due, Joseph Merrick could be remarkably vague about the details of his personal life. He was even uncertain about his year of birth, recording it as 1860 in the pamphlet, the *Autobiography of Joseph Carey Merrick*, which is reproduced as an appendix (pages 223–4). Throughout the pamphlet the chronology is therefore haphazard and unreliable, but as we have seen, he was ten years old when his mother died of pneumonia. It was an unfortunate stage of his life for him to be deprived of her love and affection, though he was always to carry her in his mind as an idealized but vivid memory. It was a memory of someone who had seemed to him the source of all the warmth and comfort that he ever knew. For Joseph, the disaster marked the end of his childhood. It was, as he wrote, 'the greatest misfortune of my life . . . peace be to her, she was a good mother to me'.

The widower Joseph Rockley Merrick now clearly faced a number of difficulties. He was left with the task of raising two young children while combining his duties as engine driver at the factory with the running of the haberdashery shop. He could not have turned to his own parents for help, for his father was dead by now and his mother had herself needed to find work in the cotton factories to make ends meet. He therefore came to a decision to break up his home and move his family into lodgings.

He found accommodation for them at 4 Wanslip Street, Leicester: a little street only a few hundred yards away from where they were living previously. Their landlady, Mrs Emma Wood Antill, was a young, twenty-nine-year-old widow who had children of her own. It was to her that the care of his own son and daughter was entrusted, and after a short interval there came about what might be seen as a predictable conclusion to this course of events: on

3 December 1874, Joseph Rockley Merrick and Emma Wood Antill were married in the Archdeacon Lane Baptist Chapel. Their marriage certificate describes Emma as the daughter of a gentleman.

For young Joseph his father's remarriage was a further calamity. Handicapped as he was by his distressing condition and his injured hip, he now found himself living in competition with stepbrothers and stepsisters who, as he said poignantly, were more handsome than he was. It was a situation that condemned him to be the odd-one-out in the new family grouping, and ultimately the family outcast. He would never succeed in gaining the affection of his stepmother, who rather seems to have made his life 'a perfect misery'. Whatever emotional response his father may have been capable of showing towards him in the past, there are indications that, within his new marriage, he became decisive in rejecting his lame, ugly and embarrassing offspring, though on two occasions his sense of duty did prompt him to go out to find him and bring him home after he had run away. It was his father's younger brother Charles Merrick, a hairdresser, who, as will be seen, became the only member of the family to find a warm place in Joseph's memories of these years.

Yet another change of address brought the family to live at 37 Russell Square, in a house attached to the haberdasher's. From here Joseph attended the newly built Board School in Syston Street until, at the age of twelve, the statutory school-leaving age established in Britain by the Education Act of 1870, he left, his education considered to be complete. The time had come when it was expected that he would go out to find work and begin contributing to the family economy. It was, of course, Emma who was particularly insistent that he should try to find work, and it was on the face of it a sensible enough view to take. Given Joseph's circumstances, however, it was to become a source of bitter and insoluble family conflict.

Having made a persistent search, Joseph eventually did find employment at the factory of Messrs Freeman's, Cigar Manufacturers, of 9 Lower Hill Street. He kept his job there for the best part of two years, but by the time he was into his fifteenth year the increasing weight and clumsiness of his deformed right arm made it impossible for him to carry out the finer movement necessary to the craft of hand-rolling cigars. He was forced to relinquish his post, and to enter into a period of long unemployment.

Each day, as Joseph tramped about the town in search of a job to replace the one he had lost, his appearance and crippled state went steadily against him. He was becoming ever more keenly aware of the financial burden which he represented to his family; he was, indeed, never allowed to forget the fact, facing the endless accusations of his stepmother that he had been idling on the streets instead of searching for employment. Often enough Emma would set his plate before him with the remark that it was more than he had earned, though the plate might be only half full. He found himself the target of sneers and jibes which wounded him so sharply that he began to avoid taking meals at home. For preference, he would limp about the streets, stifling his hunger rather than face the acid tongue of his stepmother, who made no secret of how offensive she found his presence in her household.

No doubt his father was by now in an uneasy and unenviable position, torn between whatever sense of duty remained towards his son and the shrill, strong-willed demands of his second wife. At least it may be said in Joseph Rockley Merrick's favour that he put forward one more attempt to solve the problem of employment which his crippled son was facing, even if it was to be the last such effort he made on the teenaged boy's behalf. He obtained for him a hawker's licence from the Commissioners of Hackney Carriages, and so Joseph, equipped with a tray of stockings and gloves from his father's shop, was sent out to peddle haberdashery from door to door.

It was by this stage too late for any such venture to succeed, if it could ever have hoped to do so. Each year which passed saw a steady amplification of Joseph's deformities. The mass protruding from his mouth was making his speech virtually unintelligible to strangers, and he was now so distressing a spectacle that, as he limped slowly through the streets, people would stop and turn to gaze after him. Some of the more curious might even start to follow along behind, staring at him whenever he paused. Any maid or housewife who came unsuspectingly to answer his knock at their door would invariably find the sight of him standing on the threshold thoroughly unnerving. He soon came to realize that people were avoiding answering their doors if they knew that it was he who was sounding their bell or knocker.

To support himself, meanwhile, he was expected to sell a definite quota of his goods each day. It became an increasingly difficult task. According to the anonymous article in the *Illustrated Leicester Chronicle*, the day inevitably arrived which saw his failure to sell the required quantity. Joseph, malnourished as a matter of course, spent the little money he had taken on food for himself. When he eventually returned to the house in Russell Square, he received the severest thrashing he ever was given. The blows broke more than his skin; they destroyed the last slender bonds which bound him to his father. He left the house knowing that this time he would never return.

As he dragged himself about the streets of Leicester, hawking on his own account and selling whatever goods he could, buying the small amounts of food he could afford, sleeping at night in the lowest of the town's common lodging houses, he was on the verge of destitution and little more than a vagrant. His father sought for him no more.

Joseph Merrick's uncle Charles was, as has been said, the only member of his immediate family of whom he kept a warm recollection from this period of his life. Charles Barnabus Merrick was, in fact, the youngest of the three sons born to old Barnabus and his wife Sarah. The style he established for his own life was one of well-ordered thrift and industry, for rather than follow his father into the trade of bobbin-turner at the cotton factory, he chose instead to became a barber's apprentice. It was an apprenticeship that was long and hard. He must have experienced years as a lather boy, his hands becoming sore from rubbing lather on to the sandpaper chins of customers who were shaved only every second or third day, for the cut-throat razor was beyond the dexterity of many men to use on themselves, and the services of the barber were too expensive and time-consuming to be enjoyed more than two or three times a week.

Later, as a young assistant, he no doubt practised his techniques on his father and brothers, besides learning the arts of hairdressing, singeing and beard-trimming. (The beard had returned to favour following a fashion set by soldiers in the Crimean War, when it had, during the winter months of the campaign, been too cold to shave.) Eventually, his apprenticeship completed, he married and in 1870, at the age of twenty-four, opened his first shop as hairdresser, tobacconist and umbrella-repairer at 144 Churchgate, Leicester. It was to prove a stable and well-founded business, bringing security to his family for the rest of his working life.

Yet, in spite of this security, the lives of Charles Merrick and his wife Jane were not without their troubles. By 1877, the year in which Charles's nephew Joseph found himself virtually destitute on the streets, they had seen three of their four children die before reaching the age of eighteen months. Even so, as soon as Charles Merrick heard about Joseph's plight he made a directly practical response. He went out into the streets of the city to search until he found the boy, then persuaded him to go back to the house in Churchgate above the hairdressing saloon. He and his wife would take his nephew into their own home to be treated as one of the household.

Joseph continued to hawk haberdashery about the town, but now he enjoyed at least the security of knowing that he had a place to return to where he would be offered understanding and practical support. It was a period of his life which lasted for another two years, and they must have been years of relative happiness, apart from the fact that there was no remission in the merciless advance of his condition. His peddling expeditions did not grow any more easy. It now became the usual thing, whenever he ventured out, for a small crowd to collect and follow in his wake wherever he went in the streets. In the end, his appearance attracted so much comment and attention that the Commissioners for Hackney Carriages, on the grounds that they were acting in the public good, felt obliged to take action. When Joseph's hawker's licence came up for renewal, the commissioners withdrew it.

In this way an arbitrary fate once again deprived Joseph of a means to a livelihood, and he can have had few illusions about the chances of his finding any other. In his uncle's household, the extra unproductive mouth to feed, which he unwittingly became, could only have placed considerable extra strains on the family finances. Besides, his aunt was expecting a further child. He could not expect to continue as such a burden in these or any other circumstances, but his choice of action was now in effect non-existent. He could only seek the co-operation of the Poor Law authorities and apply for admission to the Leicester Union Workhouse.

He spent the days over the Christmas period of 1879 with his uncle Charles and his family in the house above the shop in Churchgate. The heartache may be easily imagined, but during the last few days of the Old Year, still aged no more than seventeen, he parted from the only living members of his family to have treated him with charity and decency and threw himself on the mercy of the parish.

On the first Monday after Christmas 1879, a morning uncomfortable with showers of rain and a southerly wind, Joseph Merrick presented himself to Mr William Cartwright, relieving officer for the No. 2 area of the city. The Board of Guardians responsible for administering the Poor Law in the parishes of the Leicester Union in fact employed two relieving officers. William Cartwright was the junior of them, but his work was nevertheless responsible and difficult. He was answerable for his actions not only to the Board of Guardians who were his paymasters, but also to the law. While expenditure on relief work was stringently supervised and regulated by the Board of Guardians, it was the relieving officer who remained liable to be summoned to court to face charges should he commit the misdemeanour of refusing relief in a case where legal entitlement existed. Should a destitute person be denied relief and subsequently die, the relieving officer concerned might even face an indictment of manslaughter. For carrying out his duties, William Cartwright received the salary of £45 a year.

When Joseph presented himself, demonstrating his deformities and pleading an inability to work, Mr Cartwright can have found little difficulty in reaching his decision. The necessary order authorizing Joseph's admission

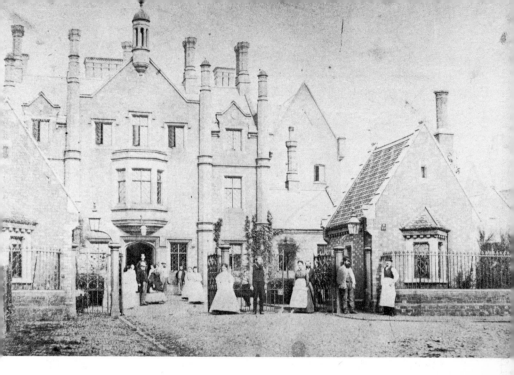

Plate 18. The Leicester Union Workhouse in the 1850s. Joseph Merrick was first admitted there in 1879

to the workhouse was issued at once. So it was that same morning that Joseph dragged his lame leg and disconcerting body up the gentle rise of Swain Street, through the grey puddles of Sparkenhoe Street to the Leicester Union Workhouse.

We may be sure that the routine of his admission was a miserable enough business. The establishment stood on rising ground, on the south-eastern outskirts of the town. It consisted of a complex of large red-brick buildings, each having three or four storeys of closely spaced and small square windows. The design of the building was monotonous and nondescript, typical of the Victorian workhouse style. Only the main building, standing immediately within the gates and flanked by two gatehouses, possessed a touch of monolithic individuality. It presented a high façade of Victorian Gothic architecture, and its great central front door had square, ornate headings. A relatively tiny, rather quaint oriel bow-window pushed itself out from the front of the building immediately above the door, while tall, thin columns of brickwork, two on either side, ascended vertically to end in little mock turrets high up amid a cluster of graceful chimneys. But the overall effect remained heavygoing, and uncompromisingly authoritarian in intent.

Presenting his pass at the gates, Joseph was escorted to the admission block for the ritual of registration. He gave up his clothes after the pockets were searched, any money found in them being confiscated as a contribution towards his keep. His own clothes were put away for when, if ever, he might be discharged. The workhouse clothes then issued to him were made of heavy serge or fustian, drab in colour and undistinguished in pattern so as to make it seem that the inmate was wearing a kind of uniform. Before he could dress himself in them, however, he would have been put through the ordeal of the 'hot' bath. (A Leicester journalist who once disguised himself as a tramp so as to sample the amenities of the Union ferociously recorded the bitterly cold water into which he was forced at this stage of his escapade.)

Ultimately, there was the entry that needed to be made in the workhouse register. This large brown book, with its list of admissions and discharges, has been preserved in the archives of the Leicester Museum; and it faithfully records the admission of Joseph Merrick on Monday, 29 December 1879, giving his name and parish correctly. The year of his birth is curiously given as 1861, but this, as has been seen, was a matter on which Joseph remained habitually vague throughout his life. His religion is described as 'church', his occupation as 'hawker'; the reason for admission is stated as being 'unable to work'.

Beyond the main admission block, pathways threaded their way between the tall, barrack-like buildings, passing workrooms, labour yards, kitchens, storerooms, laundries, until, at the very back, they opened out into the workhouse yards. Here plain wooden benches stood in the shadows of the towering buildings, and the high, encircling wall shut out all but the grey wet sky and the wind. To step through any of the doorways was to step into a world of echoing stone corridors and draughty stairways that Joseph, with his lameness, must have found hard to negotiate. There were the communal dining halls, and there were high dormitories where the beds stood close together, thin cotton sheets and drab blankets covering straw-stuffed mattresses. As they brought Joseph to show him his typical bed space, with its own small locker for his personal belongings, he was looking down at the only corner in the vast complex of buildings which he might undeniably call his own.

To comprehend something of Joseph's life during the few years in the workhouse, it is necessary to understand something of the principles underlying the Poor Law administration. Workhouses were never intended to be pleasant or comfortable places; they were meant to solve the problem of deciding which of those among numerous applicants for aid were genuinely in need, and which were not. The Poor Law Amendment Act had proposed that, as an alternative to 'outdoor relief', given as food or money and usually a matter of only a few shillings at a time, the applicant for assistance should be offered the shelter of a workhouse. Here all his or her needs would be supplied, but life would be hard, regimented and in general discouraging to anyone who was not truly in a state of destitution. For such a policy to work, the workhouse existence needed to be made at least a degree less attractive than the life of the most lowly paid labourer. In many nineteenth-century parishes, rural as well as urban, such an ideal of harsh austerity must have been no easy thing to achieve.

The Board of Guardians of the Leicester Union of Parishes first erected their workhouse in 1838, designing it to accommodate 400 paupers. Yet they remained reluctant to apply the 'workhouse test', as it was called, in all its severity, and continued to give outdoor relief on a large scale. Unfortunately, the hosiery trade, on which the town depended, then entered into a series of depressions. Unemployment became widespread until, in one period during 1848, the board found themselves paying relief to 19,000 people out of a population of 60,000. To their horror, they discovered they had disbursed over £19,000 in six months. Reluctantly the Board of Guardians decided to apply the 'workhouse test' more generally, but before this could come into force the workhouse itself needed to be enlarged. In 1851 it was rebuilt to accommodate 1,000 souls.

On the day when Joseph Merrick was admitted, there were 928 inmates in occupation. All were classed as paupers, but the circumstances which forced each of them into the workhouse varied greatly. Some were elderly, no longer able to fend for themselves; some were widows left without means of support; some were sick and infirm. Then there were the workmen, brought to poverty by unemployment or a sudden recession in their trade; the craftsmen forced to sell their tools before becoming eligible for admission; and the wives and children of these destitute men. Homeless, unmarried mothers would also be admitted to the workhouse for their lying-in. Orphans and abandoned children, tramps and vagrants, improvident paupers, even the mentally retarded and unsound of mind, also sought refuge there.

At the workhouse gates this unhappy tide of humanity was segregated into groups, according to age and sex. Husbands were parted from wives, children from parents, boys from girls, toddlers from infants. Each group went into the separate blocks, to live apart, work apart and exercise apart. Only at mealtimes or in chapel might there be a chance of a fleeting glimpse or a few snatched words.

Joseph fell within Group No. 1, of adult males between the ages of sixteen and sixty. This was the group which most concerned the workhouse authorities: adult males who had somehow failed to support themselves. Joseph's companions were thus the broken workmen, the drunkards and dissolute, the inadequate and handicapped, the crippled and retarded. Association with the frankly demented he was spared, since Leicester possessed its own separate system for the insane.

His life was controlled by bells, from the waking bell which rang as early as five or six in the morning. All other main events of the day – meals, work and rest periods – were signalled by bells. At ten in the evening, the doors of dormitories were locked and gas-lamps extinguished. Inmates were forbidden to go outside the workhouse or receive visitors unless they obtained a written order from one of the overseers beforehand. They were allowed neither beer nor tobacco. Their food was basically nutritious, but plain and monotonous, and it suffered from the hazards that almost invariably afflict institutional cooking. There were even dishes which seemed to be inventions unique to the workhouses, such as the oatmeal gruel referred to in some establishments as 'hell-broth'. Only at Christmas was the boredom of meals temporarily dispelled. To mark the festive season the Board of Guardians at Leicester customarily issued an instruction 'that the usual Christmas dinner of beef, pork, plum pudding and beer be served to the inmates of the workhouse'.

Plate 19. Pauper women eat dinner in the St James's Workhouse in the London Borough of St Pancras, *c.* 1900

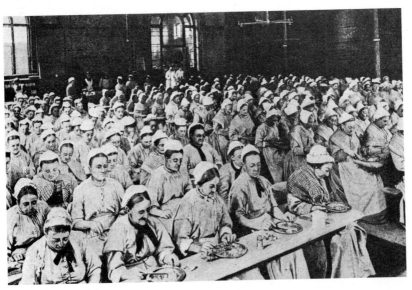

Petty breaches of discipline were punished by restriction of diet or loss of privilege. The refractory offender, defined as one who transgressed twice within one week, might find himself confined alone for one day or two. Such serious offences as refusal to work or striking an officer of the institution could lead to an appearance before the magistrates' court and a subsequent prison term. The workhouse, indeed, lived up to its name. None were allowed to remain idle. About its grounds stood the labour yards, sheds whose interiors had been divided into stalls so that a man might work undisturbed by his fellows. One of the most common among a range of thankless tasks was that of oakum-picking, the beating and unravelling of pieces of old rope and rag into a loose hemp that could be used again. It was awkward, tiring work, made more clumsy by the fact that many of the mallets provided at Leicester had lost their handles. At the end of each work period, the beaten hemp would be carefully gathered and weighed, for there was always a work quota to be accomplished. Other inmates would have to meet a quota for wood-chopping, corn-grinding or the breaking of granite into chips for use on the roads. There was also digging to be done on the workhouse allotments.

Plate 20. Pauper men at table in the Marylebone Workhouse, London. This and Plate 19 illustrate the dead weight of regimentation which governed the lives of the destitute

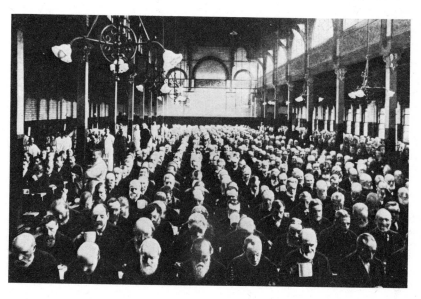

For women, there was perpetual washing and cleaning, but the hours of drudgery were long. Six and a half hours of washing was considered to be the equivalent of picking three and a half pounds of oakum. There was also the mending and making of workhouse linen and clothing, as well as work in the kitchens and dining-rooms. For the elderly, there were the duties of supervising the infants or the boys and girls, acting as helpers in the lying-in rooms or as nurses for the sick, or even taking charge of the mentally retarded. For the younger children, there was the workhouse school where epidemics of minor eye infection caused the Leicester authorities recurrent concern.

Only for the infants was nothing arranged, but then, as late as 1905, a Royal Commission inspecting workhouses was distressed by the provisions it found for the care of infants in many institutions. It spoke with justifiable concern of young babies lying unchanged in cold, wet cots; of babies who had no hope of getting outside into the sunlight and fresh air, the only attendant present having no means of carrying them all down several flights of stairs from the nursery to the ground floor; of the helplessness of a single attendant faced with the task of feeding a roomful of toddlers from a bowl of rice pudding while armed with only one spoon.

Yet, hard as conditions were, they provided basic standards of shelter and as often as not were comparable with the conditions of home life that many inmates had known. There were even families, 'the ins and outs', who, to the consternation of the administrators, seemed to flout and even exploit the whole 'workhouse test' system by thriving on the existence. These would sign themselves in during times of need, and out again whenever there was a race meeting, fair or market being held in the vicinity.

At the outset, Joseph Merrick endured the workhouse routine for twelve weeks, but then, on Monday, 22 March 1880, he signed himself out, putting on his own clothes again and leaving shortly after breakfast. For two days he sought for work, but found only that his circumstances were unchanged. On the evening of the second day he was forced to turn once more to the relieving officer for help. On this occasion it was the senior relieving officer, Mr George Weston, who interviewed him and evidently heard his case sympathetically. He was granted a further order for admission, but it was too late to return to the workhouse that night, and only on the following morning did he present himself at the gates. The same ordeal of admission and registration awaited him, though now he managed to give the year of his birth correctly, and his religion as that of his mother, 'Baptist'. The reason for admission was recorded as 'No Work'.

It had been a last, hopeless protest against the inevitability of his pauperism. Now he must resign himself to this existence, to a life that he would later speak of with loathing and horror. On this occasion his workhouse term would last unremittingly for a full four years. We can only guess at the humiliations he is likely to have suffered, at the petty tauntings which his condition must have attracted from both staff and fellow inmates in an institution that was not meant to be anything but heartless.

About half-way through his workhouse years, probably in 1882, but the exact date is uncertain, one episode did occur to disrupt the institutional monotony into which his life had fallen. His deformities were still advancing and were causing him increasing distress. By the standards even of the workhouse he must have presented a remarkable sight, for the mass of flesh that grew from his upper jaw, and which so resembled the trunk of an elephant, was still quite literally growing. It was now eight or nine inches long and forcing back his lips so that he found it difficult to eat without losing the food from his mouth. His speech was almost incomprehensible, and it was the mass from the upper jaw, of all his deformities, that caused him most distress. In due course he was referred to the surgeons of the Leicester Infirmary for advice.

There were at that time three surgeons associated with the infirmary (known today as the Royal Infirmary, Leicester), the eldest of whom was Mr Thomas Warburton Benfield, who had come to Leicester as a young man after qualifying in London in 1843. He then held various appointments and won several distinctions, working mainly for the poor in voluntary Poor Law establishments. By the early 1880s, however, he was in a state of semi-retirement, his successor as senior surgeon at the infirmary being Charles Marriott, whose younger colleague was Julian St Thomas Clarke. All three had distinguished themselves during their training and subsequent careers, and there was no question but that they were highly qualified and capable in their field.

The Leicester Infirmary was itself a good provincial hospital; its results compared respectably enough with those obtaining in other hospitals about the country, though they were still depressing enough. As the hospital records for 1882 show, for the 587 operations performed there was a loss of only twenty-three lives – but the operations listed include many such minor procedures as the avulsions of toenails, incisions of abscesses, circumcisions, and amputations of fingers. By contrast, of eighteen hernias treated surgically, three died. Two years later, in 1884, there were nine cases which required the abdomen to be opened, and only five of these survived. Mr Benfield, in an address to the Midlands Branch of the British Medical Association, of which he was president, was able to speak proudly of a mortality rate as low as one in fourteen for operations to remove stones from the bladder, but the most routine operation could still be a perilous venture once the risks of haemorrhage, shock or hospital sepsis were taken into account.

It is possible that Joseph was seen by all three surgeons at the Leicester Infirmary, but no records survive to tell us which undertook responsibility for treating him. It was most probably Mr Marriott, since Mr Benfield was by now associated only as a consultant. At all events, Joseph was advised that something might be done to help with the swelling from his mouth, provided he was willing to take the risk of an operation. It cannot have been an easy choice, given the reality of the existing hazards, and at the best of times the average expectation of life in the 1880s was still only forty-one years. Yet Joseph placed himself in the hands of the surgeons, ready to take the risks for the relief which their knives might bring him. Arrangements were made for him to be admitted to the infirmary.

By that time the long, dark wards of the Leicester Infirmary had already witnessed a century of suffering. With its 189 beds it differed little from other voluntary hospitals of the day. For support it depended on the contributions of a host of benefactors, whose names and subscriptions were carefully recorded each year in the annual hospital report. It was administered by a Board of Governors selected from among the more generous of the benefactors. Apart from accident or emergency cases, or private patients, admission could only be obtained by a letter of recommendation from a benefactor. The number of cases which a benefactor might recommend in any one year was proportionate to the scale of his subscription.

The hospital wards were noisome places, with lines of low beds, each having its neat cotton counterpane. Pictures hung on the walls and the serpentine pipes of overhead gas-lamps ran across the ceilings. There were open fireplaces in each ward, involving the inevitable accumulations of coal dust in the hospital corridors. The centre of the ward was dominated by the ward table with bulbous brown legs and on its surface large winchester jars of medicine. There was the as yet consistently unsolved problem of fleas and bugs in the wards and cockroaches in the kitchens.

The nurses, in long dresses and starchy white aprons, stiff collars and white caps, worked long hours, as many as fourteen hours on day duty or twelve hours on nights; though two hours were free once a week, and they enjoyed one half-day and one Sunday off each month. In their first year of employment, they were paid £1 a month. Some received training, but most, particularly those of the older generation who occupied the more senior posts, had learnt their professions in a hard experience which seemed to scar their personalities with a characteristic emotional toughness and cynicism.

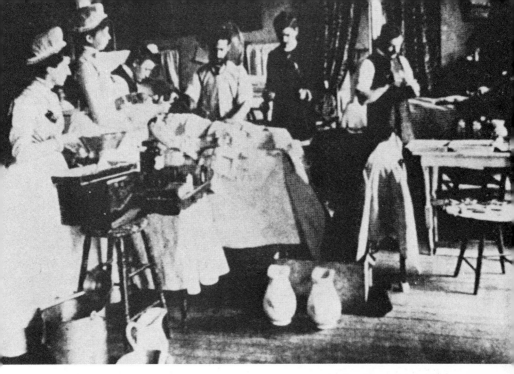

Plate 21. A surgical operation in progress in the 1880s

From what is known of the hospital routine, it is possible to reconstruct the course of events from the moment when Joseph was taken into the operating theatre. This was a large room where everything seemed to be centred on the wooden table in the middle, its hinged flaps capable of being folded away from beneath any limb to be amputated. Underneath the table rested a convenient box of sawdust. There was also a black metal box in which the surgeons' instruments were stored, white china jugs to hold hot water and an ever-present irritating smell of carbolic spray. While the nurses continued to wear their everyday uniforms, the surgeons stood waiting in their waistcoats, their sleeves rolled up as they prepared to scrub their hands with soap and lysol before soaking them in, first, carbolic lotion, and secondly, a solution of bioiodide of mercury. It was their practice to work bare-handed.

Also awaiting Joseph was an enveloping mask of cotton gauze to go over his mouth and nose, a towel to be laid over his eyes, and then the sweet pervasive smell of chloroform and a continuing but distant sense of pain and panic.

The operation seems to have been a success, for the larger proportion of the 'trunk' on Joseph's face was removed. It can only have been a terrifying and dangerous experience, but remembering it afterwards he was able to dismiss it with the words: 'I then went into the Infirmary at Leicester ... when I had to undergo an operation on my face, having three or four ounces of flesh cut away ...'

On the corner of Wharf Street and Gladstone Street, close to the Lee Street house where Joseph was born, there stood a hotel known as the Gladstone Vaults. Its proprietor was Mr Sam Torr, whose official business was listed in the *Leicester Directory* as 'Wines and Spirits Merchant and Manufacturer of Aerated Water'. In fact he was already far better known as a star of some magnitude in the British music hall, being a figure of great popularity on the London halls, including Wilton's, where he presented his song material in the style of the *lion comique* – the song defining the character role, whether comic or sentimental, and interspersed with patter. After he had made his first fortune working the London music halls, he went to Leicester, not far from his home town of Nottingham, where his father had been a tailor, and at first became licensee of the Green Man in Wharf Street.

When he took over the Gladstone Vaults, Sam Torr most certainly had his eye on the possibilities it held for being adapted into a premises with music hall attached. His ambitions had been fulfilled with the grand opening there,

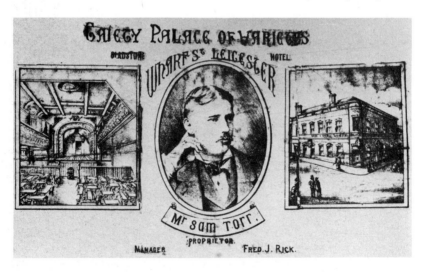

Plate 22. Advertisement for the Gaiety Palace of Varieties which Sam Torr owned in Leicester and on whose stage (*left*) he exhibited the Elephant Man

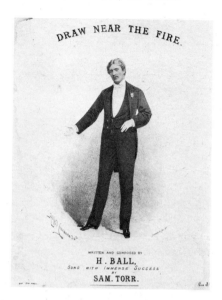

Plate 23. 'Draw Near the Fire': a Sam Torr song-sheet cover shows him singing a sentimental ballad in the pose of a *lion comique*

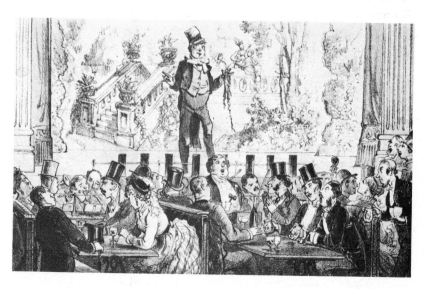

Plate 24. A typical scene in an early music hall: 'An Anti-Idiotic Entertainment Company', drawing by Alfred Concanean (1874)

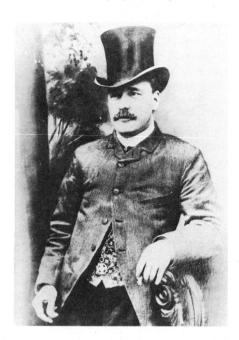

Plate 25. Sam Torr in the role of music-hall entrepreneur at the height of his career

on 3 September 1883, of the Gaiety Palace of Varieties. Top of the bill for the opening night was Vesta Tilley, 'The Masher King ... The London Idol', and among the supporting acts were Mrs John Wood, 'Nightingale of the Midlands', Mr Wilfred Roxby, 'Legitimate Character Comedian', and Messrs Young & Sandy, 'Negro Comedians'.

The hall, reported the *Nottingham Journal* on the day of the opening,

has been converted into a spacious and excellently appointed saloon for the purpose of furnishing amusement to its frequenters. A select area near the orchestra and the chairman's seat is reserved for about fifty persons. There are seats for about 200 in the body of the hall, while a promenade gallery will accommodate a similar number. The stage is admirably arranged, and in point of tasteful decoration is scarcely surpassed by the other places of amusement in the town ... evidently no expense has been spared to render the hall as attractive as possible.

It was Sam Torr's declared intention to run his establishment along 'high class lines', seeking to cater for the 'better class society of the hosiery metropolis', and the prices for admission ranged between 6d. and one guinea.

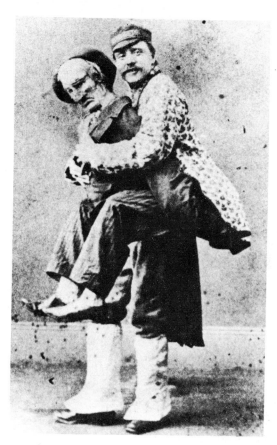

Plate 26. Sam Torr dressed to perform his speciality number, 'On the Back of Daddy-O'

The Gaiety had as its chairman Mr Will Till, himself a baritone soloist, who introduced the turns and generally presided. It also had its resident orchestra, which was coerced into performing by a lady conductor, Mademoiselle Banvard, who rejoiced in the title of 'Leader of the Band'. Its proprietor would also not infrequently appear on his own stage to sing a selection from his repertoire of comic ditties, the greatest success and constantly demanded favourite being 'On the Back of Daddy-O'. This he would perform dressed in an ingeniously devised, life-size dummy with a wickerwork frame, on whose back he appeared to be sitting while it cavorted to the music. It was a droll effect which never failed.

There were six verses to the song, the first of which ran:

> Here I am, friends, how do you do,
> They call me Sam the silly-o.
> This is my old Dad you see,
> Happy, good old Billy-o.

And each verse was followed by the chorus, sung 'in quick time whilst galloping around stage':

> Gee up, gee whoa, and away we go,
> Mind yourself old laddie-o,
> Gee up, gee whoa, and away we go,
> On the back of Daddy-o.

It has been suggested that the figure of 'Daddy-o' was the precursor of the ventriloquist's dummy of the later variety stage tradition, but while Sam Torr addressed remarks to it, he never made it speak in its own right. 'Daddy-o!', however, became a well-known catch-phrase of the day, and is said to have been as popular as 'By Jingo!' for a time in Victorian London.

In the meantime, the idea had been taking root in Joseph Merrick's mind that the one escape route remaining if he was ever to get out of the workhouse – the one hope he could ever have of paying his way in the world – might be to place himself on exhibition as a freak. He had heard that Sam Torr was interested in exhibiting specialities and novelties which might make a turn or display for the Gaiety, and it was therefore to Mr Torr that Joseph wrote. The comedian responded by paying Joseph a visit in the workhouse and summing up his possibilities.

The prospect of taking on Joseph as a property certainly caught his attention, but he was too good a showman to under-estimate the likely complications. No exhibition featuring Joseph could hope to remain for more than a week or so in any one place before its novelty began to fade. For such a plan to succeed it was essential that arrangements be made for him to travel to a succession of towns. It all needed a degree of thought and organization.

Sam Torr's solution was to set about bringing together a group of businessmen with interests and establishments similar to his own. Within a short while he was able to tell Joseph that he had managed to persuade four fellow

Plate 27 (opposite). The record of Joseph Merrick's discharge from the Leicester Union Workhouse on 3 August 1884 appears in the second line on this page of the ledger

DISCHARGED.

Date. 1834	Day of the Week	Admitted or Discharged	NAME.	1	2	3	4	4a	5	6	7	8	8a	9	How Discharged; and if by Order, by whose Order.	In case of Death, say "Dead."	Observations on General Character and Behaviour in the Workhouse.
Aug[?] 3rd	Sun	D[?]	Winn James		1											Dead	
	Mon	D	Emanuel Joseph		1										Own Request		
		D	Shingles Joseph		1										Own Request	Dead	
4		D	Whitbread William		1												
5	Tue	D	Douglas Robert														
		D	Alloy Thomas		1												
6	Wed	D	Williams John		1										Own Request	Dead	
		D	Peat Charles		1												
		D	Atkinson William		1		1										
7	Thur	D	Clark Enoch	1			1										
		D	Tollett Maria		1		1										
		D	Dent		1												
		D	Gotch William									1					
		D	Eliza														
8	Fri	D	Newbery Thomas						1		1						
		D	Wakefield Caroline									1					
		D	Pearce Horace														
		D	Lucy														
9	Sat	D	Carter Mary Ann												Fetched out by Father & Mother	Dead	
		D	Allen Mary Ann						1						Fetched out by Friend		
		D	Quinton Isabel									1			Own Request		
		D	Beaumont Mary							1					Fetched out by Brother		
		D	Medford Archie				1								Do		
		D	Thomas												Do		
		D	Henry														
			Carried Forward	1	8	1	7		4	1	3				2	26	

managers to come in with him to form a syndicate to organize Joseph's exhibition as a freak. As a result, on Sunday, 3 August 1884, Joseph was able to eat his last institutional breakfast, reclaim his clothes, go through the formality of signing himself out and turn his back on the Leicester Union and all other workhouses for ever.

It was an interesting group which Sam Torr brought together to manage the promotion of Joseph's new career. Besides himself there was one other music hall proprietor: Mr J. Ellis, who styled himself 'the Caterer of Public Novelties' and owned The Living, a Palace of Varieties at the Bee-Hive Vaults, Beck Street, St Anne's Well Road, Nottingham. Two members of the group were travelling showmen who specialized in the exhibition of freaks, the first of them being Mr George Hitchcock, known familiarly in the circles in which he moved as 'Little George'; and the second Mr Tom Norman, who has already been met with and about whom more will shortly be learned. Last though not least there was 'Professor' Sam Roper, the founder of Sam Roper's Fair, which toured regularly out of Nottingham, across into Lincolnshire and eventually to north Norfolk and King's Lynn.

Immediately after his release from the workhouse, Joseph came under the care of Mr Torr and Mr Ellis. They prepared him for his first exhibition, suggesting that he be presented as 'The Elephant Man, Half-a-Man and Half-an-Elephant'. So far as is known, Joseph's début before the public was made at Nottingham in The Living, Mr Ellis's music hall. He was also shown in at least two other towns, including his home town of Leicester, according to one account, and there was a trip on the fairground circuits with Sam Roper. The time came, however, for the partnership to cast its eyes on the possibilities of the great metropolis, London. Few knew the tricks of the showman's trade there better than Tom Norman.

It is perhaps too easy to see nothing but degradation in Joseph being forced to uncover his bizarre body to the public's gazings and ill-informed wonderings. Yet, short of a miracle, there had been for him no other conceivable line of escape from the grinding limbo of workhouse life, which could only spiral ever downwards to end in the unmarked shadow of a pauper's grave. Whatever humiliations fate may still have had in store for him, it must have been for Joseph a time of hope such as he cannot have known for many years as he took the road south with Mr Norman. It boded well to hold the key to his financial independence, the one condition which could be in harmony with his natural interior dignity. For the moment Tom Norman was the nearest Joseph Merrick came to having a fairy godfather.

CHAPTER 6

The Silver King

Of his parents' family of eighteen sons and daughters, Tom Norman was the eldest and, as he put it himself in his unpublished memoirs, on which this account is based, 'the most roving and rackety of them'. He was born in Sussex, a well-to-do butcher's son, and from early on he helped in his father's business, spending his mornings in the shop and afternoons at the local National School. At the age of twelve he left school, and by fifteen was an accomplished butcher. He was capable of going on his own to market to select and buy cattle, afterwards driving them home to slaughter them, cut them up and sell them without further supervision.

He made his meat rounds on horseback, enlivening his days by joining up with the local hunt, the East Sussex Hounds, whenever it crossed his path, usually leaving his meat deliveries hanging in a basket from a branch on any convenient tree. Unfortunately, at the hunt he caught the eye of the daughter of his father's wealthiest customer and succumbed to the temptation of paying court to her. The result was that his father lost trade and Tom was banned from the hunt whenever the young lady was present. At length his father found it prudent to deny him the use of a horse whenever a hunt meeting was due to be held.

At seventeen, Tom left home to become assistant to a butcher in London. The shop there opened at six each morning; at eight breakfast was eaten from a bench at the back; half an hour was allowed for lunch, if trade permitted; and tea was a stand-up meal snatched between customers. By ten o'clock at night the working day usually drew to its close, though it might continue till midnight on a Saturday. On Sunday, working hours were shorter, the shop being open only from seven in the morning till three in the afternoon. Tom Norman noted how it was the custom in town for women not to buy meat for the Sunday lunch until 1 or 2 p.m. at Sunday lunch-time. Yet, despite the long hours and hard work, he was contented, earning as much as 30s. a week with board and keep on top, and there was a half-crown bonus in a good week.

After a year, Tom temporarily abandoned the butcher's trade, determined to make his fortune by gambling on horses. After losing all his savings in the space of two days at Ascot, he abandoned the enterprise and set out to walk back to London, pausing only to ask his way from a stout gentleman whom he encountered in Windsor Great Park. A few yards further on he was accosted with respect by onlookers who were anxious to know what the Prince of Wales had said to him.

Back in London, he settled in Chapel Street, Islington, undertaking work as a commission agent and auctioneer in the 'live and dead' meat trade. There now occurred one of those random incidents which can unexpectedly change the direction of a life. The shop next door in Chapel Street was leased to a showman who exhibited various freaks and novelties to the public. The initial amused contempt with which Tom Norman observed his neighbour's activities became transformed into a thoughtful respect when he saw the steady stream of visitors entering the shows each day. He joined one queue and paid a penny to see 'The Only Electric Lady – A Lady Born Full of Electricity'. He watched the sparks being drawn from various parts of her body, and was startled to receive a distinct shock when he touched her hand.

It did not take much reflection to convince him that someone with his quick-witted talents – 'a man with some capital and perhaps brains' was how he phrased it – might find a great future in such a business. Within a few days he made his decision to finish with the meat trade for good and go into a business partnership with his neighbour. Their understanding was that Tom Norman would contribute the capital while the showman made available his knowledge of the business.

There was one disappointment in store for Tom Norman: his discovery that the 'Electric Lady' was a fraud. She was connected to a lead from an induction coil, the other lead being attached to a metal plate which lay under a dampened carpet on which the customers stood while viewing her.

The first exhibition presented by Tom Norman and his new-found partner was at Kingston-upon-Thames, and whatever it featured it was a wash-out. By the end of the first evening they had taken precisely twopence. Tom soon realized he had struck an expensive bargain, but he was, as ever, quick to learn. He made the discovery that even more important than the exhibit was the technique by which it was presented.

But you could indeed exhibit anything in those days [he wrote]. Yes, anything from a needle to an anchor, a flea to an elephant, a bloater, you could exhibit as a whale. It was not the show, it was the tale that you told.

Panache and patter, the building up of the sense of expectation in any casual listeners, drawing more of them in from among the chance passers-by until you had created your crowd – all this counted for more than the material. Mr Norman also made the not unexpected discovery that he possessed an inherent talent for this style of showmanship, and within a few weeks knew he had stumbled by chance on his natural vocation.

For a time his exhibitions travelled successfully from town to town, and his unpublished memoirs contain a vivid flavour of what it must have been like to be on tour with Tom Norman. A suitable 'show shop' was the first requirement, preferably in the main street of the town being visited. While such premises were honestly hired as a rule, if times were hard the use of a shop might be obtained by guile. The way this was done was as follows. In the middle of the morning on a Saturday, Tom Norman would approach the appropriate estate agent, stating that he was acting for a new

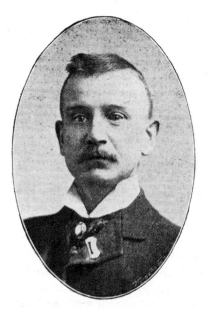

Plate 28. Tom Norman, 'The Silver King'

company which intended to open a chain of fancy bazaars. He would express interest in the vacant shop already earmarked and take the key, promising to return it on Monday morning. Since most estate agents had their own houses in the comfortable, quiet suburbs, they were not to know that no sooner had Tom Norman seen them depart safely for home at about midday than he would move into the empty premises.

In no time at all the 'props' would arrive on a small cart drawn by an old black man, who happened in this instance to be the show itself. A large canvas sheet, covered by an oil painting that bore at least a remote relationship to the entertainment about to be mounted, was then hung high up on the front of the building by a system of poles and pulleys. Tom Norman usually kept several such paintings in store, ready to be adapted for practically any class of freak. Whitening or soap was then used to write notices and 'gags' on the shop windows, sawdust was sprinkled on the floor and a large enamel Pears Soap advertisement sign was laid on the floor so that a coke fire could be lit in a bucket to heat the red-hot iron bars which the old black man would later bite and bend.

During Tom Norman's earlier days, naphtha flares were used outside his show shops, but as these grew hot, the naphtha would often begin to drip on to the pavements and catch alight so that it became a hazard to walk close by. Later, he changed to paraffin lamps, and then, when there was not enough money to buy oil for the six large lamps that were needed, the black man would be dispatched to the nearest stores to have 'three quarters of paraffin' put into each lamp. He would tell the oilman that the lamps were now too heavy for him to carry them all at once, so he would take three now and return for the others later. With the first three lamps the exhibition could be opened, and once enough money was taken the remaining three could be sent for and the oil bill settled.

When, at last, the exhibition was ready to take off, the black man, now clad in skins and feathers, with large curtain rings on his hands and legs and a ring in his nose, danced in the doorway to the shop, beating a gong or tom-tom. Tom Norman further enlivened the proceedings by telling tales of how this aged native once swam across the Orange River to save a party of shipwrecked sailors when they could not save themselves. (It was an element in the story which he hastily discarded when a knowledgeable listener informed him that anyone who wanted to could wade across the Orange River without getting their knees wet.)

With his 'touting, shouting and telling of the tale', it was not long before the thoroughfare became completely blocked by people, but it was rare for anyone to complain. These exhibitions were a common sight, and the police were usually readily persuaded to turn a blind eye, while making a habit of looking in just once during the evening, usually immediately before going off duty. Then Tom Norman, knowing what was expected of him, would slip the bobby sixpence for his trouble – always in coppers, since, he thought, it seemed a bigger sum if given in this form.

Throughout the Saturday afternoon and evening the show would continue, often staying open till midnight. It would open for a while again on the Sunday, but by daybreak on Monday the props would be safely stowed away on the cart and the show slipping quietly out of town. The key to the shop would have been pushed through the estate agent's letter-box with a note regretting that the premises had turned out to be unsuitable for the purpose the inquirer had in mind.

The shows which Tom Norman exhibited changed frequently, and he was willing to put on almost any display. The novelties which he promoted included fleas in harness, fat ladies, giant babies, tall men, short men. For a 'Savage Zulu Show' he recruited his savages from among the ranks of retired seamen living in the lower depths of the Ratcliffe Highway, and these painted themselves for the part, conversing before the customers in a gibberish of their own invention. Such shows were, of course, common enough on the fairgrounds, and it must have been one very like Tom Norman's which further inflamed the annoyance of the citizens of Northampton at the frequent mounting of entertainments on their Market Square. On 4 June 1881, the *Northampton Mercury* recorded their complaint:

> By permission of the Mayor, the proprietor of any show can pitch his tent on the Square at any time, and the latest example of the nuisance of which we are complaining occurred on Tuesday, when some Zulus were exhibited in a large booth. However estimable these gentlemen and ladies may be in other spheres, they have not proved themselves desirable neighbours in this case. During the evening they kept up a sort of exaggerated Gregorian chant, with Zulu variations, alternating with the strains of a powerful organ.

An Irish giant and an Irish dwarf, exhibited jointly as 'The Hibernian Contrarieties', made another stylish attraction, and Tom Norman also mounted the classic talking head illusion and, at a later date, even a 'wireless' demonstration, where the customers stood around the side of the room listening to music supposedly coming from London. There could be a moment of sharp disillusion in store for them should a needle stick on the gramophone in the back room.

One exhibition to which Tom Norman became particularly attached was his family of midgets. It consisted of two midgets, billed as man and wife and always brought into town in a specially constructed miniature coach drawn by ponies. In each town during a tour he made a point of closing the show down for a few days, to allow the lady midget to 'give birth to her baby'. A new-born infant would then be hired to stand in for the hypothetical offspring, and he found that even larger queues always gathered after such a 'happy event' to see the new arrival in the family. The only trouble was the difficulty he had in restraining the 'mother' from swearing volubly, smoking her pipe and drinking gin in front of the customers. The exhibition finally came to grief when the 'mother' ran away one night, objecting to being displayed as a woman any longer, both midgets in fact being men.

But Tom Norman's ventures rarely ran utterly aground. He developed into a past master in the art of attracting the attention of a crowd by numerous stunts and tricks. One of his favourite gimmicks was to announce that a particular show was booked to appear at some future illustrious event – and at this point he usually invoked the name of P.T. Barnum, American proprietor of 'The Greatest Show on Earth'. It was a trick he tried once too often. One afternoon at Arcadia, held in the Royal Agricultural Hall, Islington, he boldly stated his usual claim, only to find he had set off unrestrained merriment on the part of three gentlemen in the audience. After the show, when introduced, one of them turned out to be no less a personage than the great showman himself. Barnum then stretched out a hand to touch the festoons of Mexican and American silver dollars which Tom Norman habitually wore suspended from his watchchain, and said to his friends with wry amusement, 'The Silver King, eh?' It was enough: from a moment of acute embarrassment Tom Norman characteristically salvaged triumph. He retained the nickname until the end of his days.

As his business ventures prospered, so he found it possible to move into permanent premises. The first shop which he took over was in the Edgware Road, but by the end of six months he was proprietor of thirteen other exhibition shops in and around London. He had a 'money-taker' at each, while he himself spent his time going from shop to shop to gather the takings, watch the progress of various displays, make minor adjustments to shows and move exhibits between premises.

He was now continually short of suitable novelties and freaks, and would go to immense pains to obtain new live showpieces, often making a long train journey on the strength of a friendly tip. Having come across a suitable subject for display, he would employ a skilful guile in his approach, often spending several days in gaining the confidence of the person concerned before making a proposal. In speaking of the money he paid them, he was

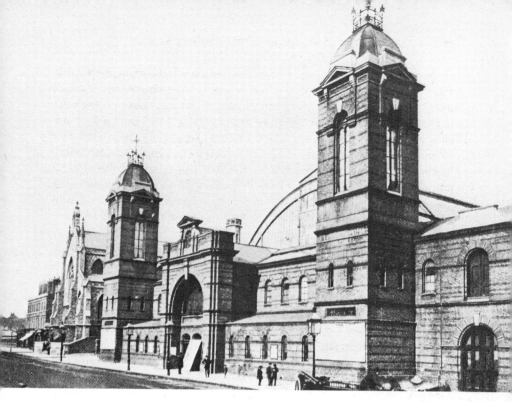

Plate 29. The Agricultural Hall, Islington, where Tom Norman met P.T. Barnum (reproduced from *Round London*, 1896)

apt to use phrases like 'star artist amounts' or 'princely salaries', and he claimed to have paid his living exhibits amounts 'that enabled them to enjoy every reasonable luxury of life'.

Should anyone level at him the charge that he was exploiting his freaks for personal profit, he defended himself by pointing out that his freaks were earning more than they could hope to do by any other means available. Besides, so long as they remained under his care they were no longer a burden on relatives or the community. He insisted that their lives as exhibition freaks were both varied and interesting, whereas the only real alternative they had was to be shut away in the dull seclusion of their homes or a workhouse. Nothing could have shaken his conviction that, for the most part, his freaks led happy and contented lives, or that he was offering them a positive alternative. While the Poor Law remained on the statute book, he had an unanswerable point.

It was during the early period when he was building up his small empire of exhibition shops in London that Tom Norman heard of Merrick, the small but grotesquely deformed young man from the Leicester Workhouse, and so became a member of the consortium which Sam Torr brought together to promote Joseph as a professional freak. The London circuit was clearly Tom Norman's area of responsibility in managing Joseph's display, and he probably did not foresee any special difficulties at this stage, especially not in the East End where the most extreme novelties found a ready and unsqueamish audience. In this way the two of them arrived together in London just three months after Joseph's release from the workhouse, and went to the small, desolate shop in the Whitechapel Road; and while they were there the events described in the opening chapters of the present book occurred.

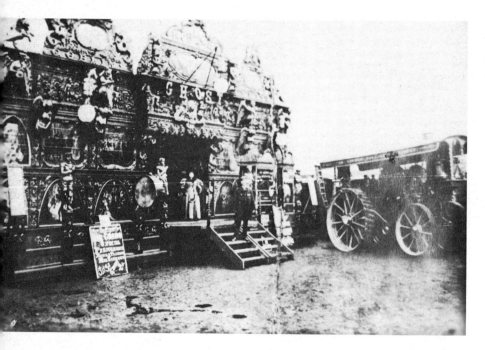

Plate 30. Tom Norman stands on the steps of his 'Ghost and Goblin Show' in a damaged but rare print

Plate 31 (opposite). The baroque fairground splendour of Tom Norman's 'Ghost and Goblin Show' can be seen more clearly in this photograph, taken at the Humberstonegate Fair, Leicester

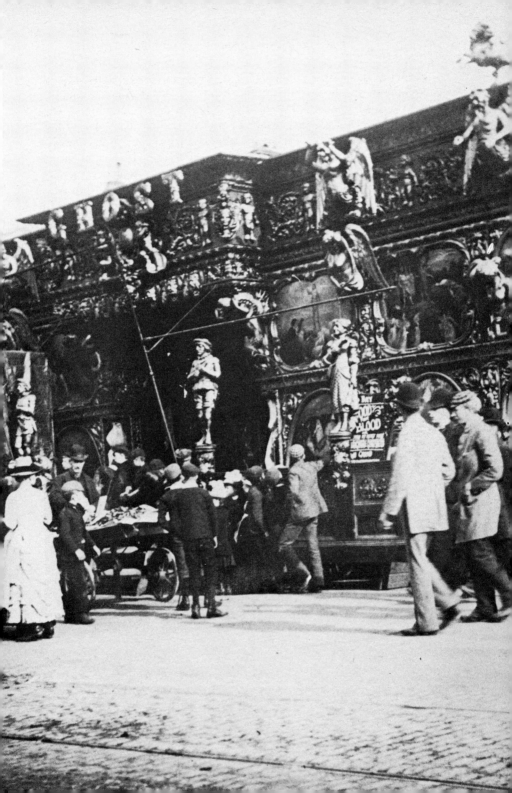

The worst that anyone could find to say about Tom Norman was that he could be a bit of a rascal, but never less than an engaging one and always a positively rough diamond. He could be disarming, even charming, in self-criticism, as when he remembered as an old man the 'very flash appearance' which he had cultivated in his youth with his curly-brimmed bowler hat, his waistcoat jingling with watchchains and silver coins and his white gloves with ostentatious rings worn on the outside of them: 'always appearing to be up to the thousand pounds a year mark, and perhaps, if the truth were known, I did not possess a thousand pence . . . I often think that my flashness proved to be a big asset.'

The contrast of the man as he showed himself to be with the surly, harsh image briefly conveyed by Frederick Treves in the opening passages of 'The Elephant Man' is, once again, striking. Norman was most emphatically no fly-by-night nonentity, but a man who knew his trade inside out, lived intensely by his wits and founded a fairground dynasty which continued in business in the British Midlands until recently. He was known as one of the most enterprising of the English showmen, having been a pioneer (the second in the world, it was said) in the use of electric light on the fairgrounds, and one of the first to adopt steam traction engines. In 1890, he also set up as a showman's auctioneer with great success, acting for such famous personalities as Lord George Sanger and the Bostock family, who had, of course, at an earlier stage, taken over the running of Wombwell's Menagerie.

CHAPTER 7

A Travelling Life

When the police closed down the exhibition shop in the Whitechapel Road, it could hardly be argued that they were acting in Joseph Merrick's best interests, but then that was not what they had in mind. They were responding to the shift in public opinion which was demanding a tightening up on the standards of what should be considered fit for public viewing. The forces of respectability were making a determined onslaught.

Joseph, back on the road in the early months of winter, can have gained little enough from his encounters with Frederick Treves and the Pathological Society of London. There was no explanation offered for his illness, no hint of a possible helpful treatment. The only souvenirs which he evidently carried away were Treves's visiting card and a set of the photographs which Treves had had taken. That this was so is indicated by the fact that one of the photographs was used as the basis for the illustration on the front of the pamphlet, *The Autobiography of Joseph Carey Merrick*, which was offered for sale to freakshow patrons.

It therefore seems that, after he left London, Joseph returned to Leicester, where the pamphlet was duly prepared and printed. There is room for some debate as to whether he actually wrote it or whether it was written for him. On this point anyone who reads it must make their own judgement, but on balance the tone and content, the words and phrases chosen, have an authentic feeling. Joseph most probably was its author, even if he did write it under the tutelage of Mr Torr or his resident copywriter. The fact that he gets his own birth date wrong may itself be seen as a slight confirmation of his authorship since, as we know, he rarely got it right. In the drawing on the cover there is also one striking detail of artistic licence: the artist has drawn in the proto-'trunk', the extension of flesh which once protruded from the upper jaw but which the surgeons at the Leicester Infirmary had already removed.

The pamphlet looks as though it was intended to be part of the promotion for the next stage of the career of the remarkable freak, and Mr Ellis and Mr Torr took the chance of advertising their respective music halls on the back. As a rule, the proceeds from the sale of pamphlets like this one went to the freaks concerned, so it may be assumed that its sale helped to augment Joseph's earnings from the music halls, show shops and fairgrounds.

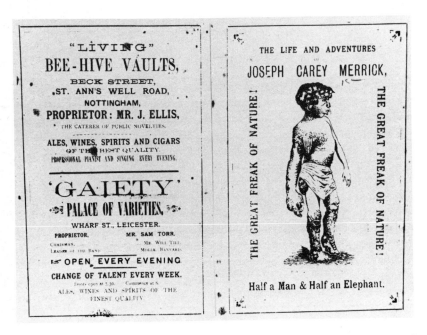

Plate 32. The back and front cover of the pamphlet prepared by the showmen which contains Joseph Merrick's autobiography

Yet, apart from the indignity of being a public exhibit, there is no reason to think that Joseph's life on the road was either unremittingly harsh or lacking in friendships. When he travelled with Sam Roper's Fair, he was given his own little caravan to journey in and hence enjoyed that degree of privacy. He was befriended on the fair by two young men who worked in the exhibition boxing booth and who were billed as 'Roper's Midgets'. Their names were Bertram Dooley and Harry Bramley. Bertram was a nephew of Sam Roper's by marriage and Harry was his cousin. William Dooley, Bertram's son, who was himself, as a professional illusionist, a top-of-the-bill performer on the music halls under the stage name of Benson Dulay, remembered his father's stories about the Elephant Man – stories which had become a tradition in the Dooley family.

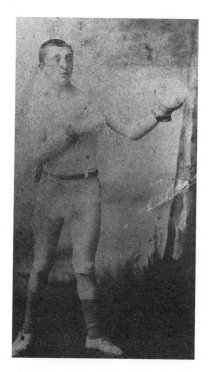 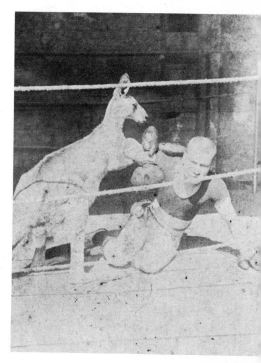

Plate 33 (*above*). Bertram Dooley, dressed for the boxing booth as one of 'Roper's Midgets'

Plate 34 (*above right*). Harry Bramley, Bertram Dooley's cousin, in the ring with the boxing kangaroo

Plate 35 (*overleaf*). Mop Fair at Stratford-on-Avon in the 1900s presents what must have been a very similar scene to the country fairgrounds where Merrick was shown

Plate 36 (*inset overleaf*). 'Professor' Sam Roper

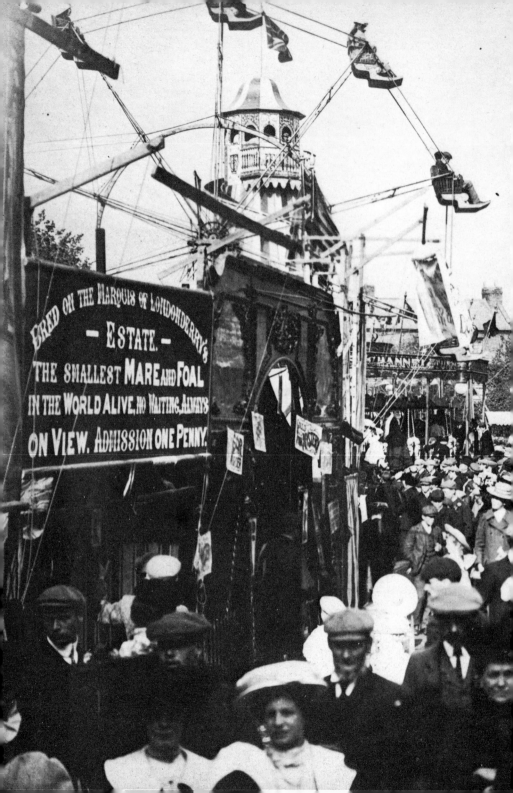

BRED ON THE MARQUIS of LONDONDERRY'S
— ESTATE. —
THE SMALLEST MARE and FOAL
IN THE WORLD ALIVE, No WAITING, ALWAYS
ON VIEW. ADMISSION ONE PENNY.

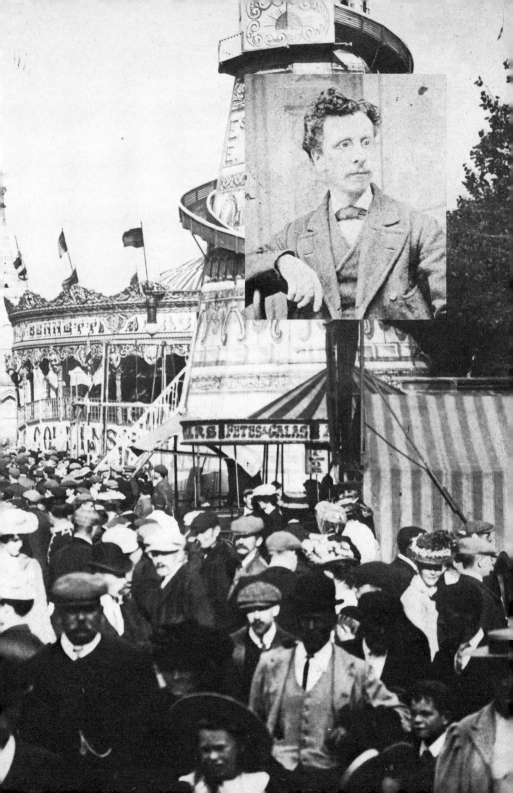

Bertram Dooley and Harry Bramley were in the habit of standing by to ward off any unwelcome attentions which Joseph might attract. Bertram used to make a point of visiting Joseph in his caravan to make sure he was all right, and would sit and talk to him there. He was impressed by Joseph's standard of conversation: 'A most interesting man – he would talk on subjects that you would never really think a man in that condition would talk about. Very upstage subjects, you know, and he was a bit on the religious side, too . . .' As for the outdoor garb and the theatrical cloak which had so taken Frederick Treves's attention when he first saw it: 'Uncle Sam thought of that, because the kids used to wait for him outside the fairground and follow him to the place where he slept.'

On one occasion, when the fair was set up on Market Square, Northampton, Joseph was harassed by a group of town lads. The ringleader took hold of the cloak to try to pull it away, but Harry Bramley, standing by, lost no time in coming to the rescue, 'and laid the boy out, completely out. He must have hit him hard, but he was a good boxer, was Harry. He was a pretty broad, well-built chap, and he could use them . . .'

The turn taken by events in Whitechapel Road, however, with the show being closed down and moved on, had been a portent for the future. Sam Roper began to grow nervous about the way the Elephant Man was drawing the attention of local officialdom. The show was being kept under close observation, and Sam began to fear that some sort of court case might actually be pending. The shocked reactions ('Oh, what a horror! What a beast!') of the viewing public must have remained consistent, and possibly the idea was spreading that Joseph could represent a health hazard and that children especially ought not to be exposed to any risk of contact.

Perhaps the main problem here was that, as a freak, Joseph was almost too great a success. The showman's patter was designed to excite the imagination and wondering anticipation of the crowd. Like the comedian's joke, it was the way it was told which made it work. And the way it was told helped to create the shared illusion with the audience which was all a part of acknowledged technique in the showbusiness, as the old-timers called their profession. The trouble began when the audience actually set eyes on Joseph and the horror of his situation became all too immediate; and doubly disturbing if one should catch a glimpse of a living, suffering being inside the dreadful shell. The viewers had never wished to find themselves facing such a reality.

At the end of the pamphlet Joseph quoted, or more precisely misquoted, a verse from a poem by Isaac Watts (1674–1748), the English Nonconformist clergyman and poet who wrote some of the finest hymns in the Protestant heritage, two of the best-known being 'O God Our Help in Ages Past' and 'When I Survey the Wondrous Cross'. In its original form, in Watts's *Horae Lyricae*, Book Two, where it is part of a poem entitled 'False Greatness', the verse which Joseph quoted runs as follows:

> Were I so tall to reach the pole,
> Or grasp the ocean with my span,
> I must be measured by my soul,
> The mind's the standard of the man.

The variations which Joseph introduces (see page 224; and also page 229) do not alter the sentiment, and it may be that he was quoting from memory a verse that had stuck in his mind since childhood. Perhaps the words once even appeared in his mother's Baptist hymnal. In the strange and pitiful case of the Elephant Man, Isaac Watts's words made their point well, though the old hymnographer could never have imagined the circumstances in which they now became so apposite an assertion of human dignity.

Nevertheless, those who felt affronted by the sight of Joseph made their complaints known. A problem of a parallel kind was recorded by the surgeon, John Bland-Sutton: 'None would give him lodging except in an outhouse, or a stable, as if he were a wild animal.' His difficulty in keeping even moderately clean on tour in these circumstances, the continual characteristic stench of his condition, the impediment to his speech which meant that only those who knew him well could follow what he was saying, must all have combined in the effect he had on others to intensify the sense of being outcast. He can hardly have been the ideal touring companion, even though Sam Roper did provide him with his own caravan.

So far as the attitude of his managers went, Tom Norman was forthright in his protestations:

> I can honestly state as far as his comfort was concerned whilst with us, no parent could have studied their child more than any or all the four [sic] of us studied Joseph Meyrick's ... The big majority of show-men are in the habit of treating their novelties as human beings, and in a large number of cases, as one of their own, and not like beasts.

Nevertheless it does not take much imagination to feel that living in close proximity to Joseph must have imposed peculiar limitations and tensions. On the other hand, one of Tom Norman's boasts that he certainly made good was that the showmen were acting in their exhibits' financial interests as much as their own. During the period of his exhibition, which Tom Norman stated was not above thirty months (it could, in fact, have been no more than twenty-two), Joseph managed to accumulate savings of about £50 from his share of the takings and maybe from some income from the pamphlet. At a time when whole families might have as little as £1 a week on which to subsist, Joseph was thus able to put aside between 10s. (50p) and 12s. (60p) a week. His £50 was an appreciable nest-egg, sufficient to maintain him without working further and in reasonable comfort for a year at least. He was quietly affluent, far better off than ever in his life before, and better off than many of those who crowded into the freakshows to view him.

But the difficulties were hardly evaporating with time. The opinion that freakshows were nothing more than exploitations of the afflicted continued to gain ground. Those who possessed civic responsibilities came more and more to see it as their duty to clamp down on all these and similar social evils wherever possible. Within the bounds of the City of London itself, the tightening up was already achieved and the exhibition of monstrosities and freaks was a feature of the past. Beyond the City's limits, in the sprawling inner suburbs, the display shops still flourished, for here authority lay in the hands of a diversity of overlapping parish and borough councils. With such a confusion of local governing bodies, any uniform policy was impossible.

The East End, with its teeming working-class population, had long held special attractions for the showmen. There always had been freakshows in the East End, and the exhibitions of monstrosities and prodigies were, as has been seen, daily events in the Whitechapel and Mile End roads. Yet even here there were changes in the air, and few were more shrewdly aware of them than Tom Norman. It was being proposed that the various London parishes and boroughs should be amalgamated into a single, giant authority, the London County Council. In only three years' time, the Local Government Act of 1888 would make this union an accomplished fact, and the newly formed authority would spring into vigorous action, bringing social reform into every corner of people's lives. Within a few months all the freakshops would be swept away, and Tom Norman, his small empire destroyed, would find himself having to adapt to a life of touring in the provinces.

I well remember [he wrote] an old showman telling me of the change about to take place, and, 'Tom,' he added, 'when it does, your and my occupation is gone.' As far as the show shops are concerned, he was right. Those that do not believe me, just test it in one shop alone. Why you would get closed up, before you got open.

Already, in 1885, the cold draught was being felt in the freakshow business as police and magistrates became steadily more persistent, more determined in their opposition to the exhibition shops. For the showmen, any exhibition which might attract both the attention and the opposition of the police was becoming a less and less desirable property. The crux of the matter was that fate had brought Joseph Merrick into his chosen profession a little too late.

It is impossible to say exactly when the decision was taken to send Joseph on a tour of the Continent. The reasons for it were obvious: to avoid the increasing harassment of the English police and to go on show in countries where the police and the authorities might be expected to be more relaxed about these matters. Perhaps it was also the case that the novelty value of the Elephant Man was wearing thin on the circuits available to Sam Torr, Sam Roper and the consortium.

One reliable source states that the manager who took over Joseph Merrick's interests on the Continent was Austrian. William Dooley, on the other hand, remembers his father saying that it was an Italian with a name like Ferrari who proposed the tour – 'an Italian born, but he was really the same as a cockney Italian, like the ice-cream version, and Sam Roper got talking to him, and "Oh", he said, "I will put him in a show like yours, and I am going on the Continent", and he took the Elephant Man away from us, which Uncle Sam didn't mind really. He didn't want to lose him, but at the same time he felt there was something there for him, you know, and Ferrari took him away with him on to Belgium . . .'

Unfortunately for the foreign showman and his new property, the police forces of Europe proved just as resistant as that in England to the exhibition of Joseph's deformities. The tour was a failure from the beginning, leading Joseph ever more closely to disaster. The police continually moved on and forbade the show, and after a number of months of shifting from place to place, it became clear to the manager that he had little hope of making any gain on the venture; that he had landed himself with a dead proposition.

In early June 1886, the shadowy figure of Mr Ferrari finally abandoned the Elephant Man in Brussels, compounding his villainy by stealing the £50 which Joseph had managed to save. This was how Joseph awoke one morning to find himself abandoned and destitute in a foreign city where he had neither friends nor hope of assistance, and where he was totally unable to communicate with those about him. For any normal person it would have been an unpleasant enough situation, but for Joseph it was catastrophic. His predicament was extreme, and his one thought can have been somehow to reach England again. With difficulty he pawned the few possessions he had left, raising barely enough to pay for his passage home.

Frederick Treves's account in his essay is unfortunately far too condensed to be much help in disentangling the course which events now followed.

The impresario, having robbed Merrick of his paltry savings, gave him a ticket to London, saw him into the train and no doubt in parting condemned him to perdition.

His destination was Liverpool Street.

The point has already been made that Joseph's savings of £50 were far from paltry by the standards of ordinary working people, and one only wishes that his journey to his home country could have been the relative plain sailing which Treves implies. The element of guesswork remains ever-present, but the facts are as follows. In 1886 the established cross-channel route from Brussels to England was by way of Ostend and Dover, the Hook of Holland terminal familiar to modern travellers not being established until 1893. There was an alternative route to Harwich, and hence to Liverpool Street, but this went round by way of Rotterdam, a long way to the north and a far longer and more expensive journey. The through ticket from Brussels to Liverpool Street is therefore unlikely. It would make far more sense for Joseph to have made his way to Ostend in the hope of the regular packet service for Dover, which would in due course have delivered him into London at Victoria Station.

It is, indeed, at Ostend that we next have news of him, but the saga of his journey home was already entering into its most miserable phase as he travelled on the train from Brussels. To his own consciousness, inside his poor distorted skull, in an advancing state of bewilderment and panic, it must have seemed to Joseph that he was on the road to his final crucifixion. The faces of strangers, who spoke in languages he could not understand, pressed themselves against the carriage windows and gaped in attempts to catch a look beneath the great hat's veilings. If he descended from the train, the crowd mercilessly followed after his bizarre and shuffling figure which-ever way it tried to turn. At Ostend, a blow as savage as any other fell when the captain of the cross-channel ferry, appalled by Joseph's appearance and mindful of the feelings of his passengers, refused to give him passage.

That he turned out to be not entirely friendless in Ostend even in these circumstances was one piece of good fortune which he certainly deserved. 'I have had the most awful case in my care at Ostend,' wrote Wardell Cardew to the well-known actor of the day, W.H. Kendal, in a reference to the Elephant Man. It has not been possible to trace the identity of Mr Cardew, but he seems to have been someone with at least medical connections who was able to offer Joseph the help and shelter he so desperately needed. Perhaps it was on his advice, with the change of plan now forced on him, that Joseph would have next made his way back north along the coast for sixty miles to the leading Belgian port of Antwerp. From Antwerp the regular packet service to Harwich was well established. It had been in operation since 1864 and worked as a branch of the Great Eastern Railway.

By 1886 the service was daily except Sundays, the run being shared by three 'railway' steamers. The senior ship of the team was the paddle steamer *Princess of Wales*, built in 1878 but joined in 1883 by a pair of ships, the S.S. *Norwich* and the S.S. *Ipswich*. These were the first Great Eastern Railway packet ships to be propelled by twin screws rather than paddles. They were handsome vessels, designed to carry both cargo and passengers, and each was 260 feet in length and round about 1,050 tons in gross weight. Their hulls were long and low, their superstructures unobtrusive, and on each a pair of tall, narrow funnels was raked at a distinctive angle.

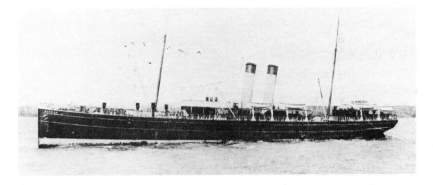

Plate 37. The S.S. *Norwich*, one of the three 'railway' steamers which was making the crossing between Antwerp and Harwich at the time when Joseph Merrick returned from the Continent

The precise date of Joseph's embarkation for home is not known, so we cannot say which of the three packet steamers gave him passage. The second-class fare from Antwerp to London, however, was 15s. (75p) at this time, and it must have taken the last remnant of Joseph's money. At least on this occasion he succeeded in passing muster at the gangplank and getting himself aboard. The departure time from Antwerp was at 17.00 hours each evening, so the long 150-mile crossing of the North Sea took place mostly during the hours of darkness. Joseph must have spent the night passage suffering from cold and hunger out on the decks, seeking a spot where he might merge into the shadows, sheltered from both wind and the eyes of fellow passengers.

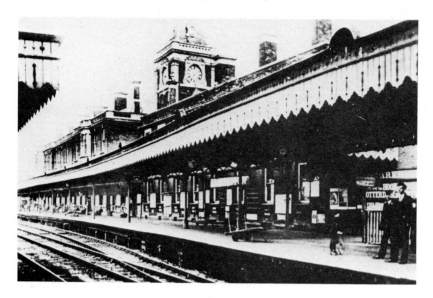

Plate 38. The platform at Parkeston Quay station where Merrick would have boarded the boat train to Liverpool Street

Plate 39. This Great Eastern Railway boat train ran between Harwich and the Midlands, but is of the same type and rolling stock that would have carried Merrick to London

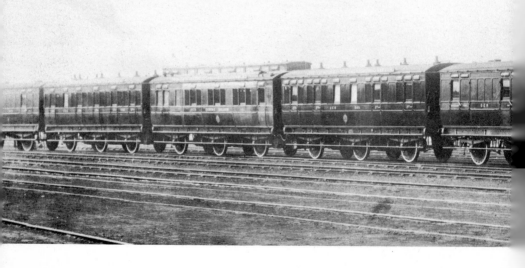

Docking time at Harwich came shortly after 4 a.m. As he shuffled wearily along the boat train in the disorientating light of early dawn, searching for a carriage where he might sit in isolation, Joseph perhaps felt a momentary sense of relief. At least he had regained the relative sanctuary of his own country. At 5 a.m. the final stage of his journey began when the train pulled out of Harwich to carry him over the last sixty-five miles to London. Its scheduled time of arrival at Liverpool Street was ten minutes to seven.

Did Joseph sleep away the journey, or were his thoughts coherent enough for him to turn over the problems which now faced him? They were surely immense, and to all appearances insoluble.

For several days he had been travelling towards a destination that did not really exist beyond the end of the tracks at Liverpool Street Station. His resources were expended, his energy exhausted. What the next step should be was a question which found no answer. Circumstances had deprived him of the last remote hope he had of paying for his keep in the world; his only security, his savings, were stolen from him. Liverpool Street was for him a metaphorical as well as a physical terminus. Joseph Merrick's destiny had finally and utterly been taken out of his own hands.

It is unlikely that Sam Torr, Tom Norman or Sam Roper could have been of much help to him by this stage. His value as a novelty had worn thin and the moral opposition was a formidable barrier. In any case, Mr Torr had his own problems, the response in Leicester to the 'quality' music-hall fare with which he attempted to provide the town having been disappointing. The

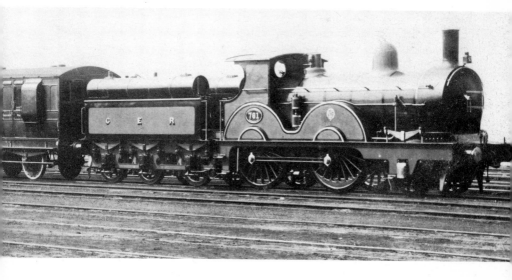

Gaiety at the Gladstone Vaults was closed by now, pending new management, and Mr Torr was back in London, picking up the threads of his career
as a *lion comique* on the halls.

Strangers who were approached by Joseph recoiled in horror and revulsion
and made no attempt to understand the broken speech which came from his
lips. There was no hotel or lodging house which would receive him; no café
or restaurant which would serve him; no hospital that would accept him as
a patient, for he could not share a public ward nor pay for a private one, and
his condition was in any case regarded as incurable and untreatable. Only at
a workhouse might he demand admission, and even there he would be
eligible, as a transient vagrant, for no more than a single night's stay. The
next morning he would be obliged to pay for his lodging by labour in the
work sheds before being turned out to walk on the thirty miles or so to the
next workhouse or 'spike', for vagrants were never allowed to stay two
consecutive nights in any one Poor Law institution unless it was the one
which served the parish in which they were accepted as resident. Only at
Leicester would the Board of Guardians seriously consider letting him become a permanent charge on the rates. And Leicester lay ninety-eight miles
away from London, even supposing he could summon the strength to walk
such a distance; and in the knowledge that once the doors of that terrible
place closed again behind him it would this time be for ever.

When Joseph Merrick finally, inexplicably, appeared on the platforms of
Liverpool Street Station amid the steam, smoke and bustle of a Victorian
railway terminus speedily awakening into early-morning life, it was as it
always had been for him, only worse. His will was gone, his demoralization
complete, and the attention which his figure drew to itself was instant,
whether he tried to move on or stood stock-still. The crowd gathered with
its usual murmuring comments, the fingers pointed, the eyes stared. Early
travellers paused, wondering what was starting the commotion, and the
crowd grew, acting as a magnet for the newcomers who pressed ever closer
in their attempts to gain some kind of glimpse.

It was the police who stepped in and forced back the by now highly
excitable crowd, guided the helpless, terrified and extraordinarily top-heavy
little figure into the haven of the third-class waiting-room; then held the
doors of the waiting-room against the press of people who clamoured to be
let in for a sight of the strange being which had come among them. Freed
from the buffetings of the human storm outside, Joseph at once collapsed
into the furthest and darkest corner of the room. The policemen who leaned
over the evil-smelling and huddled bundle could make nothing of the high-
pitched, run-together words which it tried to utter. They saw only that with

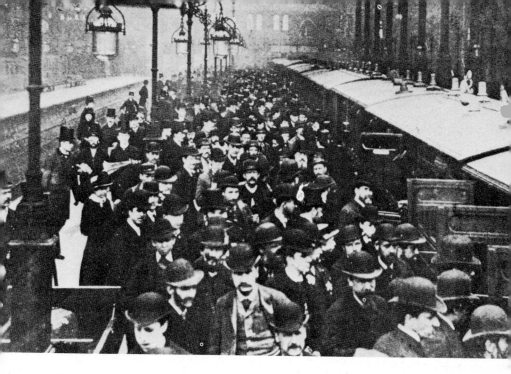

Plate 40. A crowded platform at Liverpool Street Station, illustrated in the *Railway Magazine* (December 1898)

its one evidently uncrippled hand it fumbled in an interior pocket and brought out a small oblong of much-thumbed pasteboard which it offered.

The police inspected the card. It had on it the name of a gentleman apparently connected with the London Hospital, and they knew the London Hospital well enough. It was not much over a mile away, and the place to which every victim of an attempted suicide or murder, every unfortunate who was injured in a street accident or fight would be referred on that side of London. The gentleman should be sent for to see what advice he could offer or what light he could throw on this odd, disturbing traveller.

Frederick Treves's morning's work at the hospital can hardly have begun when the message arrived, asking if he would be willing to go to assist the police at Liverpool Street Station. When he arrived, the crowd about the waiting-room was still so thick that the surgeon had some trouble in pushing his way through. As at length he managed to get in at the door and to enter the waiting-room, the figure of the Elephant Man was immediately recognizable to him. It was huddled close against the wall as if trying to shrink away to nothing. Treves realized that his former acquaintance must by now have passed beyond the limits of endurance and be completely broken.

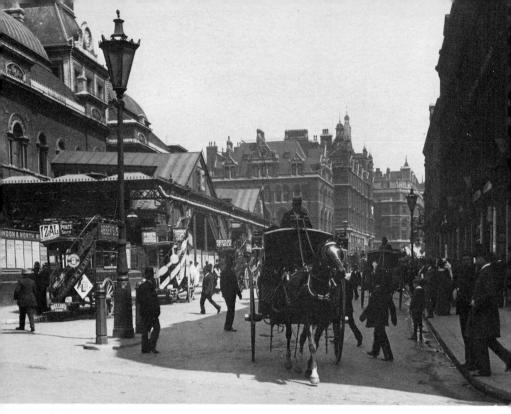

Plate 41. The scene outside Liverpool Street and Broad Street stations when the traffic was still horse-drawn

After a few words with the police, the surgeon agreed to take responsibility. With their help he then shepherded or half-carried the staggering Joseph out through a crowd to where a hansom cab was waiting. They bundled him in, and instructions were given to the driver as Treves himself clambered into the confined interior. The Elephant Man questioned nothing, but sat in a silent daze, seemingly all at once overcome with a great, trusting sense of calm. Then, as the cab turned out of the station, he sagged into a sudden and astonishingly childlike sleep.

As they clattered through the streets, Treves, sitting in the cab filled with the well-remembered stench of Joseph's body, must have begun to consider the implications of the responsibility he had accepted. The righteous system by which society sought to control the lives of the poor and destitute could offer Joseph nothing to meet his true needs. At best they might shut him away in the anonymous harshness and squalor of an institution to await his death and so erase himself from the world's consciousness. The rules themselves were founded on the Protestant ethic at its most perverse: that material prosperity represented the natural reward of virtue. Joseph and those like him had no business to exist.

Frederick Treves's mind was already made up that the time had come for the rules somehow to be broken, and he was prepared to use his own prestige to that end. Having descended in his hansom cab like a *deus ex machina* to rescue a broken life, he intended to see the role through to the end.

The hansom cab, with its incongruous pair of passengers, returned to the London Hospital, and Joseph was helped to a small, single-bedded isolation ward, tucked away up in the attics. Here he was washed, given food, put to bed, and for the moment left to sleep and dream.

There was only one brief disruption to his new-found peace and quiet when a nurse bringing food, and not forewarned of what to expect, came through the doorway and saw the figure of Joseph for the first time. The tray she was carrying crashed with its contents to the floor as the woman screamed and ran off down the corridor. But Joseph, propped up exhausted against his pillows, seemed too weak to notice the commotion.

CHAPTER 8

Come Safely into Harbour

It was a little short of six months after Joseph Merrick's unorthodox not to say irregular admission to the London Hospital when readers of *The Times* opened their copies on Saturday, 4 December 1886, to find a letter that was attention-catching even within the strongly individualist tradition of that newspaper's correspondence column. It was written by Mr F. C. Carr Gomm, the chairman of the London Hospital management committee, and in effect it launched an appeal, not on behalf of any fund for medical relief or general charitable cause, but for an individual. The uniqueness of the circumstances certainly needed to be well defined for such an appeal to be justified. It began:

Sir,
    I am authorized to ask your powerful assistance in bringing to the notice of the public the following most exceptional case. There is now in a little room off one of our attic wards a man named Joseph Merrick, aged about twenty-seven, a native of Leicester, so dreadful a sight that he is unable even to come out by daylight to the garden. He has been called 'the elephant man' on account of his terrible deformity. I will not shock your readers with any detailed description of his infirmities, but only one arm is available for work.

In the paragraphs which followed, Carr Gomm outlined the Elephant Man's history: how, some time before, Mr Treves, one of the hospital surgeons, saw him on exhibition. How the police stopped the exhibition and Merrick went to Belgium under the care of 'an Austrian manager', who left him robbed and destitute. How he pawned his last possessions, which raised his fare to England, where he felt that 'the only friend that he had in the world was Mr Treves of The London Hospital'. How the crowd had made his journey home an utter nightmare, and how when he arrived at the hospital he had 'only the clothes in which he stood'.

He has been taken in by our hospital, though there is, unfortunately, no hope of his cure, and the question now arises what is to be done with him in the future.

He has the greatest horror of the workhouse, nor is it possible, indeed, to send him to any place where he could not insure privacy, since his appearance is such that all shrink from him.

The Royal Hospital for Incurables and the British Home for Incurables both decline to take him in, even if sufficient funds were forthcoming to pay for him.

Mr Carr Gomm then reviewed in detail the administrative difficulties which Joseph's case raised, but made the point that, as an incurable, he ought not to be taking up space in an already overcrowded general hospital, 'where he is occupying a private ward, and being treated with the greatest kindness – he says he has never before known in his life what quiet and rest were'. Joseph's appearance, said Carr Gomm, was so terrible that

... women and nervous persons fly in terror from the sight of him, and that he is debarred from seeking to earn his livelihood in any ordinary way, yet he is superior in intelligence, can read and write, is quiet, gentle, not to say even refined in his mind. He occupies his time in the hospital by making with his own available hand little cardboard models, which he sends to the matron, doctor, and those who have been kind to him. Through all the miserable vicissitudes of his life he has carried about a painting of his mother to show that she was a decent and presentable person, and as a memorial of the only one who was kind to him in life until he came under the care of the nursing staff of The London Hospital and the surgeon who has befriended him.

It is a case of singular affliction brought about through no fault of himself; he can but hope for quiet and privacy during a life that Mr Treves assures me is not likely to be long.

It was symptomatic of the spirit of the times that Carr Gomm found it so necessary to emphasize not only that Joseph was in no position to do an honest day's work, but also that no moral taint attached to his plight. To be utterly deserving of charity it was essential to be utterly virtuous. Oddly enough, Joseph's character did approximate to such an ideal, and many of those who met and came to know him would have agreed without argument. The fact perhaps made Carr Gomm's task of raising the appeal that much easier, and he threw open an invitation to the influential readers of *The Times* to put forward suggestions for Joseph's future, while also making it clear that there was no question of the hospital ejecting the patient on to the street, even though it was at this stage in its history having to deal with some 76,000 cases each year.

> I have never before been authorized to invite public attention to any particular case, so it may well be believed that this case is exceptional.
> Any communication about this should be addressed either to myself or to the secretary at The London Hospital.

As it happened, a complex series of perplexities and discussions had led up to the drafting of Carr Gomm's remarkable letter. Frederick Treves had precipitated an administrative dilemma into the laps of the hospital committee when he acted to commandeer the little room tucked away among the attics in the roof of the East Wing. It was one among a set of rooms that had been converted so as to accommodate single private patients or isolation cases suffering from highly infectious diseases. The very act of admission was in technical breach of hospital regulations, as Treves himself recollected.

> Chronic cases were not accepted, but only those requiring active treatment. I applied to the sympathetic chairman of the committee, Mr Carr Gomm, who not only was good enough to approve my action but who agreed with me that Merrick must not again be turned out into the world.

For the time being, however, it had been a question of ignoring the irregularities of Joseph's presence in the hospital, and Treves was free to examine Joseph at leisure. He was startled at the deterioration in physical health which had taken place during the year and a half since he last saw him. The Elephant Man presented a pitiful sight: his deformities had increased to the point where their crippling effects were becoming more general; he had also developed bronchitis, and there was at least the suggestion of a heart disorder in an early stage. Eighteen months before, at the meeting of the Pathological Society of London, Treves had been able to note how Joseph enjoyed good health, how he was free from other serious disease apart from his condition, and how he even possessed a fair degree of natural strength. Now he was driven to recognize that Joseph's expectancy of life could not be more than a few more years at the most.

After his admission to the London Hospital, Joseph's general condition remained poor for several days, but gradually a combination of food and rest helped him to recover some of his lost strength. The problem of the stink which arose from his skin was resolved more easily than might have been expected, for it was found that so long as he bathed once or twice a day, the odour could be reduced to a level that was hardly noticeable. It was also arranged that he should be attended only by nurses who volunteered, and that each of these should be carefully prepared for his appearance before being admitted to the room. In this way the usual shocked reactions of people seeing him for the first time were avoided.

He remained, even so, a difficult patient to nurse. His speech was almost incomprehensible, and he showed suspicion towards anyone who approached him. It was becoming clear that his spirit had suffered even more than his body from his recent experiences. Every knock on the door of the room, Treves noticed, would provoke a reaction of startled anxiety. He would flinch from the hands of his nurses, and he shook with agitation whenever a stranger entered his room or whenever some thoughtless, sensation-seeking wardmaid or porter pushed the door of the room ajar to take a peep through the crack.

For the course of many days Joseph remained unsettled and apprehensive, but at last the steady routine of hospital life and a growing familiarity with the doctors and nurses who attended him soothed his shattered nerves. He settled into a cautious, watchful repose. He began to form tentative friendships with the hospital staff, expressing a shy but deeply felt gratitude for everything they were able to do for him. His manner, always gentle, now became almost serene, and he developed a childlike faith in those who tended him. The nurses would bring him cardboard cutouts from the toy shop to help him pass the time, and together they struggled to construct the models. Each finished model would then be solemnly presented to some member of staff as a token of the gratitude which he felt but for which he could never find sufficient expression in words.

As time went on, Treves grew increasingly accustomed to the Elephant Man's odd speech, and found he was able to talk with him and study him more easily. There were fresh examinations to be made and measurements to be taken; once again Joseph was persuaded to strip and pose for the clinical photographer. At least there was for Treves, as he visited Joseph each day, the professional satisfaction of witnessing a slow return to relative health – but simultaneously there hung between them, unspoken, even evaded, the question of Joseph's future.

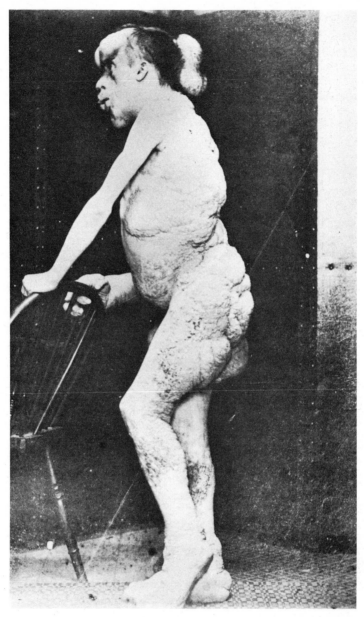

Plates 42a–d. The photographs of Joseph Merrick which were taken in December 1886 and show his condition at the time of his admission to the London Hospital

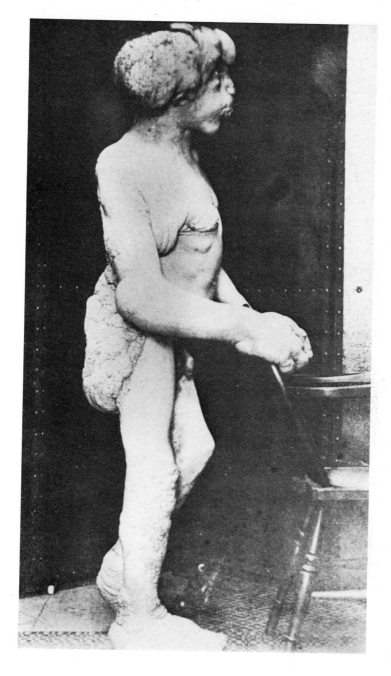

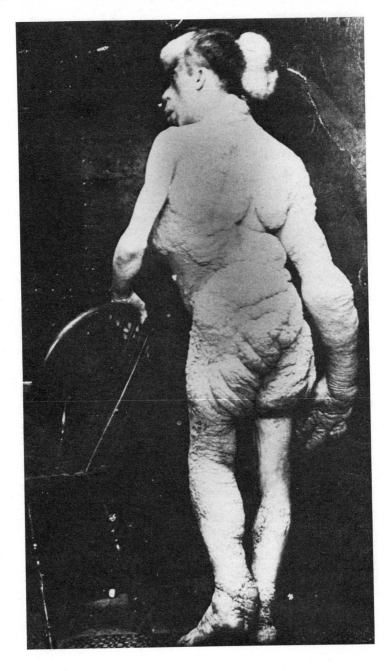

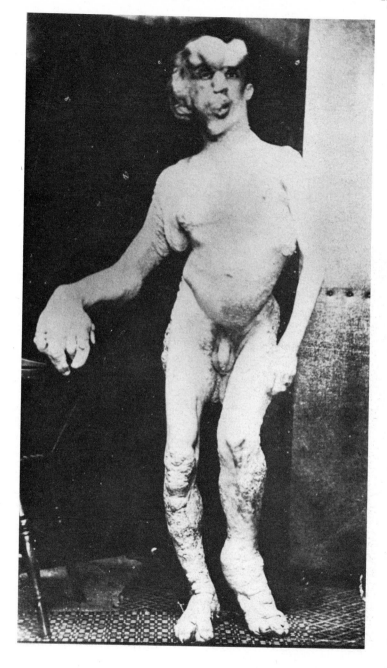

By November 1886, the blind eye of the authorities could not be relied on to remain turned for much longer. Five months had passed since Joseph's admission, and while he could still hardly be described as a fit man, it was obvious that little further improvement could be expected from the treatment the hospital had to offer. He was, moreover, occupying a private ward, urgently needed for other patients and for which no payment was being received. There were no other institutions which could be persuaded to offer him shelter, and even the hospitals for the chronic sick which Carr Gomm approached had refused to give him a place. It seemed unthinkable that he should be callously discharged into the street, yet no funds were available to maintain him in a hospital ward where, by all the rules, he was an inadmissible case. Carr Gomm felt he could go no further without the authority of the full house committee.

At this point in the history of the Elephant Man a vigorous publicity campaign appears to have been set in motion on his behalf, though by whom it was originated is uncertain. The fact remains that events moved fast, and the starting point was a strikingly appropriate sermon preached by the Master of the Temple, Dr Charles John Vaughan, on Advent Sunday, 28 November 1886. Dr Vaughan had achieved his present eminence only by living down a homosexual love affair with a pupil, which in 1859 compromised and put an end to his career as a headmaster of Harrow School.

For his sermon that Sunday he took his text from the Gospel According to St John: 'Who did sin, this man or his parents, that he was born blind?' Was his choice of text coincidence, or did he speak from a knowledge of Joseph's distress? In theory, his attention could have been drawn to the case of the Elephant Man by Carr Gomm, who was himself a barrister of the Inner Temple. If this was so, Dr Vaughan might have been expected to take a personal interest, for he also was born and spent his childhood years in the city of Leicester, where his father was vicar of the parish church of St Martin's.

Dr Vaughan's sermon, in turn, gave Carr Gomm the chance to cite it when, two days later, he took up his pen to write to *The Times*. By preaching eloquently on the text concerned, said Carr Gomm, Dr Vaughan had shown how 'one of the Creator's objects in permitting men to be born to a life of hopeless and miserable disability was that the works of God should be manifested in evoking the sympathy and kindly aid of those on whom such a heavy cross is not laid'. The letter was accordingly printed on the Saturday, and three days after that, on Tuesday, 7 December, the house committee made the whole problem of Joseph Merrick's future care the first item on the agenda of its routine weekly meeting.

As the committee minutes concisely record, Mr Carr Gomm began, as chairman, by addressing the meeting on Joseph's behalf, outlining the steps already taken and reviewing the background to the case as well as the circumstances which led to the appeal for help being made in *The Times*.

The Chairman stated that the result had been the receipt of a very large number of letters and a considerable sum of money. About £100 had been sent for his help and a Mr Singer had offered to contribute £50 yearly if Merrick were kept here. (The only other suggestions the Chairman had received were to send him to a Hospital for the Blind, to Lighthouses or to Dartmoor.)

The House Committee considered this case very carefully and it was resolved to keep J. Merrick here for the present and the Chairman said that he would communicate with Mr Singer who made his liberal offer on Merrick's behalf.

The outcome was a public response that was literally astounding, and letters continued to arrive by every post. Even the *British Medical Journal* was moved on the following Saturday, 11 December, to investigate the matter with a mixture of aroused curiosity and professional detachment:

A letter from Mr Carr Gomm, Chairman of The London Hospital, appeared last week in *The Times*. It contained an appeal to the charitable public on behalf of John [*sic*] Merrick, a man afflicted by so terrible a deformity that he cannot venture out by daylight to the garden of the hospital. Not only does his condition prevent him from being kept in a public ward or admitted into an institution for incurables, but he cannot travel even by public conveyances. Among the other experiences of this kind, acutely painful to his feelings, a steamboat captain refused on one occasion to take him as a passenger.

The journal went on to dispose of any idea that Merrick suffered from elephantiasis, and reminded its readers that he had already featured in notices of the meetings of the Pathological Society of London, and that the case was then fully reported in the society's *Transactions*, a plate also being featured.

Since that plate was taken the disease has made great progress. Through the kindness of Mr Treves, we have been supplied with four photographs, representing the patient's present condition. A comparison of these drawings with the plate above noted will show how the disease has advanced during the past two years . . .

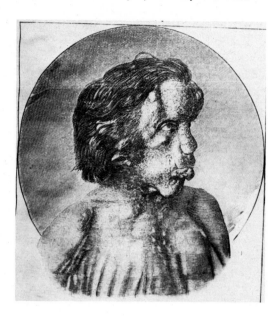

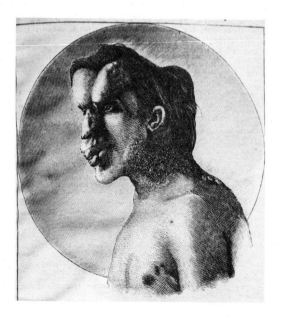

Plates 43a-b. The engravings for Merrick's head which appeared in the British Medical Journal for December 1886

We learn from Mr Treves that he has received piles of correspondence from the curious and from the charitable on the subject; and we trust that poor John Merrick will, through the efforts of the benevolent, be enabled to end his days in peace and privacy, with a small competence.

The report in closing rounded off with a rather technical discussion of Joseph's deformities, and there can be little doubt that it was inspired by Treves himself. Not only did it acknowledge his help, but it also contained the curious mistake which was the hallmark of all his writings on the topic of the Elephant Man: the erroneous statement that the Elephant Man's Christian name was John. Whereas the hospital authorities, Carr Gomm and the editor of *The Times* managed without trouble to record him correctly as Joseph, Treves invariably and persistently referred to him as John Merrick.

So far as the disposal of Joseph's future was concerned, however, the situation was beginning to grow much clearer – was, indeed, happily resolving itself – by the next appointed meeting of the hospital committee on Tuesday, 14 December. The reverberations from the letter in *The Times* stirred up responses in many other newspapers, and these in turn took up the story. The plight of the Elephant Man was even carried in the provincial press, and reached, it seems, the hairdresser's saloon in the back streets of Leicester where Joseph's uncle Charles Merrick pursued his modest, hard-working trade. A 'very great number of letters had been received about Joseph Merrick', Carr Gomm was able to tell the hospital committee,

> ... and a very large sum of money upwards of £230 had been sent to him. No useful suggestion had been made for the best means of providing for the unfortunate man, save that his uncle had offered to take him in, but it appeared that there was an obstacle to this in the necessity Merrick was under of frequent bathing. Thus a considerable sum of money had been received, and as one gentleman, Mr Singer, had given £50 which he proposed to continue annually, it was the Chairman's opinion that the best course to pursue was to keep Merrick here. This course was agreeable to Merrick himself, and although he was not strictly admissible it seemed that it was the right thing to keep him here.
>
> In this opinion the Committee unanimously agreed and the Chairman undertook to write to *The Times* announcing that his letter had been adequately answered.

It would be impossible to grudge Joseph his luck at last in the genetic destiny which had besieged his life from its beginning. He had suddenly caught the imagination of the British public in a way that could not have been possible while he remained a grotesque, disturbing showpiece in the freakshops. Only six months before, it had seemed impossible to visualize any future for him, beyond the inevitability of his being drawn down into Victorian England's insatiable and nameless maw for the destitute and broken in spirit. He also had the advantage of being the perfect object for philanthropic attention: utterly blameless and hence unqualifiedly deserving.

He had entered into his refuge.

Once it was all settled that Joseph should remain as resident in the London Hospital, it was essential for suitable accommodation where he could live to be set aside and prepared. At the back of the hospital, between the high buildings of the East Wing and the new Grocers' Wing (so called because its building had been made possible by a generous donation from the Grocers' Company of the City of London), lay the sunny, echoing courtyard known colloquially as 'Bedstead Square'. It was christened thus because it was here that the iron bedsteads from the hospital wards were brought for repair, cleaning and repainting. On one side of the square, a flight of concrete steps led downwards from the courtyard to a small, wooden door with a grimy overhead fanlight. Behind the door, bare and unused in the basements of the East Wing, were situated two small rooms. It was decided that these could make an ideal conversion for the Elephant Man's future home.

The task of overseeing the adapting of the rooms fell to Mr William Taylor, chief engineer to the hospital. He was in his early fifties, having come there in 1878 as an employee of the engineering firm which installed the lifts. Once the contract was completed, he was invited to stay on as a member of the hospital's engineering team and to help ensure that the lifts continued to work satisfactorily. Gradually he rose in rank to become chief engineer, acquiring with his post the resounding title of 'Mechanical Engineer in Charge of the Artisan Staff'.

As a consequence of Mr Taylor's labours, the larger, outer room in Bedstead Square was furnished as a bed-sitting room. There was in it a bed, a table and chairs, a small fireplace with its own mantelpiece and a pleasant armchair to set before it. The room gathered daylight from glass panels set within the door, from the fanlight above and from a narrow, deep-set sash window that looked on to the alley and the flight of concrete steps. On the inner wall of the room another door opened into a passageway, beyond which lay the second, smaller room of the suite. Here Mr Taylor managed to contrive a bathroom for Joseph's use. There were no mirrors in either room; it was the one firm stipulation which Frederick Treves laid down in the matter of furnishing.

The removal of Joseph to his new quarters was easily accomplished, but convincing him that the rooms were truly his for as long as he needed them turned out to be a more difficult undertaking. It was all so much more than he had or could have hoped for. At a stroke he was provided with the sanctuary he had been seeking ever since the first occasion when he ran away from home. The small basement rooms brought him a degree of privacy beyond his dreams. Their very remoteness from the general life of the hospital gave him security.

Plates 44a–b. The exterior and entrance as they are today to the rooms in Bedstead Square which were once Joseph Merrick's home

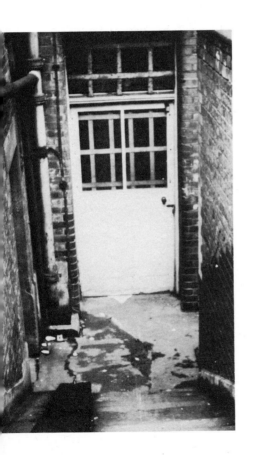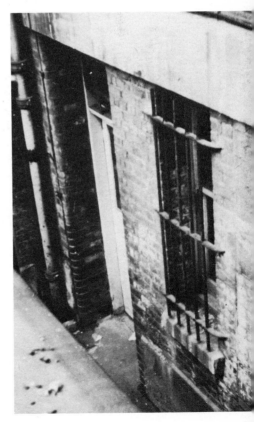

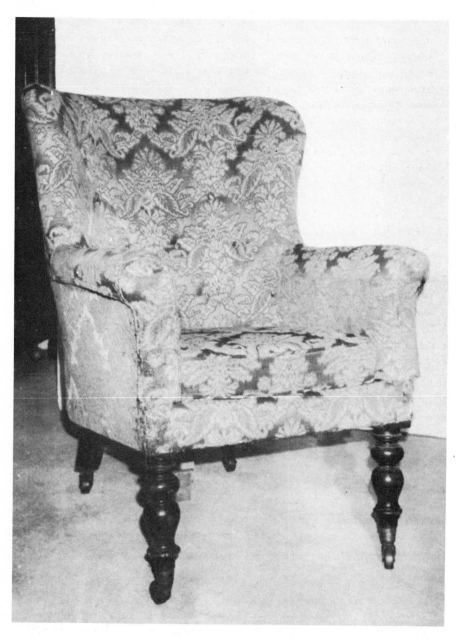

Plate 45. Merrick's armchair

He surveyed them with an air of wonder, but his good fortune was too bountiful for him to be able to grasp it all at once. He could only accept it with bewildered surprise and a barely comprehending gratitude. Meanwhile, with Joseph finally settled in quarters of his own, Treves in no way relinquished his care of his patient. He made a point of visiting him each day, and instructed his house surgeons to follow his example.

The position of house surgeon was a six-monthly appointment, and the honour of acting in this capacity was much sought after by newly qualified doctors, despite the fact that it was an unpaid labour, involving many long hours of work in the general wards, receiving room and operating theatre. Among these many chores, the visit to Joseph was not always regarded as the easiest of routine tasks.

One of the first of the young doctors to find himself undertaking the duty was Wilfred Grenfell, a student of Treves who eventually achieved fame as Sir Wilfred Grenfell of Newfoundland, where he worked as a doctor attached to the Christian missions among the great fishing fleets of those days. In his autobiography, *A Labrador Doctor*, he wrote of the period when the Elephant Man came under his care, recording how Joseph was exceedingly sensitive about his appearance and yet pathetically proud of his normal left arm. He felt that in spite of everything, Joseph managed to keep up a cheerful disposition, and described how he would speak freely as he speculated on how he would look preserved in 'a huge bottle of alcohol – an end to which in his imagination he was fated to come'.

Grenfell attempted to measure the Elephant Man's hat, but found that his arms could not reach about its circumference. He also recorded how, in due course, the accommodation in Bedstead Square came to be called 'the Elephant House'. 'Only at night could the man venture out of doors, and it was no unusual thing in the dusk of nightfall to meet him walking up and down in the little courtyard.'

Dr Tuckett, who was responsible for Treves's initial visit to the Elephant Man, similarly remembered from his tour of duty the intense pride which Merrick took in his good arm. He also spoke of his love of beauty, his great gentleness of character and the fascination which fine clothes held for him. He thought as well that he would probably have been quite a good-looking young man if it had not been for his frightful disability.

Someone who found that visiting the Elephant Man had more to it of duty than of pleasure was Dr D.G. Halsted, who held the appointment in 1887 and whose own book of memoirs, *A Doctor in the Nineties*, was published as late as 1959. He seems to have found that Joseph had a consistently dispiriting effect on his own state of mind. In the patient's features he could make out nothing of the suggested resemblance to an elephant; rather he felt that the deformed face was more like that of a tapir, 'but I suppose a "Tapir Man" would not have been such a powerful attraction as a sideshow'. He could never bring himself to see Joseph as anything but a pathetic figure, but he would try to cheer him up if he found him miserable and depressed. He confessed that he always felt happier when, duty done, he slipped away to other responsibilities.

While Treves continued to pay at least one visit to the basement rooms each day, it also became his habit to spend a couple of hours in Joseph's company each Sunday morning. He deliberately set out to study and cultivate an understanding of his patient, and grew fluent in interpreting the distorted speech uttered by Joseph's lips. It was therefore inevitable that he should become the person most closely acquainted with the Elephant Man. On Joseph's side, the pleasures of educated conversation were a new experience, and he seized on them eagerly. It was as though there existed in him a passion for talking which had lain dormant for lack of comprehending company, and now his every Sunday morning would pass in a pleasant haze of chatter with Treves.

At the time when he carried out his first clinical examination two years before, Treves's assumption was that Merrick was to some extent imbecilic. It was an impression fostered by the trouble Joseph had in giving outward sign to inner feelings. His facial deformities prevented him from forming any expression, either of pleasure or grief, and the movements of his limbs were so clumsy that any gesture had lost all spontaneity by its moment of completion. Only by a use of words was he able to convey his thoughts, and since his speech was as distorted as his mouth, his genuine intelligence and awareness tended to go unrecognized.

In the early days of their conversations, Treves tried to manoeuvre Joseph into talking about his past, but here he encountered many gaps and odd reticences. ('It was a nightmare, the shudder of which was still upon him.') There were undoubtedly areas of trauma in Joseph's remembrance of his early life, and walls of silence which Treves never succeeded in breaching, despite their special relationship. While Joseph was willing to acknowledge that he came from Leicester, he would never talk of his childhood there. He gave Treves the impression that he knew nothing whatsoever of his father; neither did he mention his sister, Marion Eliza, nor his dead little brother, William Arthur. Of his mother he did speak a little, but his description of her was so surrounded by a romantic and idealized glow that Treves firmly believed it to be only an elaboration of Joseph's deeply wounded imagination.

Joseph would talk of his mother as being beautiful, and his most precious possession remained the small painted portrait of her which he carried with him everywhere and had managed to preserve through many vicissitudes. When Carr Gomm was first shown the picture, he sensed how Joseph displayed it with pride. It was as though the picture served as a constant proof that where Joseph was himself so hideously disfigured, at least he came from undisfigured stock.

The perplexity which Joseph felt in the matter of his own distorted body was once expressed to Treves in a remark he made about how odd it was that he should be so deformed when his mother had been so beautiful. He could never speak of her without his emotions welling over, and he never actually told Treves that she was dead. It was this which led the surgeon privately to conclude that Joseph's mother must have abandoned him when he was still an infant. In fact all Joseph's memories of Mary Jane Merrick were those of a mother who had shown her crippled son a constant gentleness and unfailing love.

If he could not be persuaded to talk of his family, neither would he discuss his experiences as an exhibit in the freakshows. He did, however, rather puzzle Treves by refusing to disparage the showmen who had managed him, stressing only the gratitude which he felt towards them. His memories of the workhouse, on the other hand, invariably caused an outburst of bitter indignation. It was clear that returning to such an institution would always be intolerable for him to contemplate. Yet, in all other things, he gave the impression of looking back on his life without rancour and of accepting his misfortunes with quiet resignation. If there was bitterness at the indignities to which fate had submitted his physical body, he gave no sign.

Treves, as he listened, found himself increasingly fascinated by the world which Joseph seemed to inhabit. The ideas and opinions were often apparently curiously coloured by their owner's isolation. It was as though his disorder had forced him to become a bystander in the business of living, starving him of social relationships and of the most basic human experiences. Now all things intrigued him, descriptions of meetings, places, people, occasions; there was nothing which could not arouse in him a wistful curiosity.

As the curtains which screened Joseph's personality were slowly drawn back, Treves discovered how many of his impressions of the world came not from any first-hand knowledge but rather from books. He was an avid reader, having learnt to read as a child, and books had become a constant source of solace to him in his loneliness. His knowledge of them was both eccentric and diverse, for his selection of reading matter was determined more by whatever chance brought to hand than by consciously exploring or developing literary tastes. He had simply read anything that presented itself: the Bible and the Prayer Book several times, so that he knew both intimately. He had an extensive acquaintance with newspapers and magazines of all kinds, and even a patchy knowledge of the works of more serious novelists, including Jane Austen. He had struggled with a string of lesson books and enjoyed a host of stories. In fact he had read and considered any scrap of writing which fell into his hands, however fragmented it may have been.

Whenever he discussed his reading, the void which his books had filled and the reality they had taken on in his mind soon became apparent. He was apt to speak of novels as if they were factual accounts as opposed to fictional narratives. He would describe plots as though they were events which had happened recently, recount conversations in animated detail and speak of characters as though they possessed lives of their own, discussing their plights and predicaments with sincere concern. Through taking his books into his head, he was thus able to lead a kind of surrogate life in parallel with his own realities and to compensate to some extent for the denial to him of experiences in the real world.

At such moments, watching his excitement and involvement, Frederick Treves would realize that Merrick possessed unguessed-at emotional depths; that beneath the grave and rather hesitant courtesy lay a turmoil of emotions. Joseph could be moved to excitement and agitation, or even compassion and grief, as easily as any child, but in his case the stirring up of feelings was powerful, profound and lasting. The discovery of such fundamental and easily provoked emotions in his patient both startled and disturbed Treves.

From his reading Joseph therefore derived most of his impressions of human nature, having had few opportunities to study people closely. He had met men from many walks of life and in wide varieties of circumstance: idle sightseers, doctors, music-hall entrepreneurs, Poor Law officials, showmen, workhouse keepers, surgeons. From them he had received wide varieties of treatment and reaction, both kindly and professional, but mostly of a detached nature. His ideal of manhood meanwhile remained a strangely compounded creature. It was derived in part from novels, with their descriptions of the manly virtues of innumerable heroes, drawn, it seemed, almost exclusively from the aristocracy and living lives of idle luxury; and in part from the advertisement columns of the newspapers, with their emphases on such necessary accessories to the outward show of a gentleman as travelling bags, patent-leather shoes or dressing cases. It was a vision of the romantic hero, but as a rather demanding ideal of a gentleman it bore little resemblance to the men he had actually met.

His image of the opposite sex was even more difficult, and several degrees more intense. But his attitude to women might be defined in the most simple terms: he felt an admiration for them which bordered on idolatry. Perhaps with somewhat ominous undertones, he confided to Treves that his favourite reading consisted of stories which dealt with love and romance.

At the age of seventeen, Joseph had been admitted to the segregated wards of the workhouse; at twenty-one, he emerged into the carefully screened-off world of the showman's booth; for the past seven years, the pattern of his life had been practically monastic. Women were a complete enigma, a totally unknown quantity, and his vision of womanhood was largely an amalgamation made up from his books, his imagination and the transcending memory of his mother.

Women were thus creatures to be set apart, beings of a gentler and purer spirit. He saw each one as the heroine of some untold story, a person to be regarded with such reverence and awe that she became unapproachable, let alone obtainable. Women were and should be as they existed in the pages of romantic chivalry: delicate, more finely moulded creatures than men, needing to be protected, cherished but above all worshipped.

This was the image to which he clung throughout his life, even though it was cruelly at odds with his experience. All his encounters with women had been associated with pain and distress. Invariably in any woman whom he met there would be immediate and obvious signs of shock and revulsion. In some cases the reaction had been so extreme that they screamed and ran away, or even fainted on the spot. Only from the matron of the London Hospital, Miss Eva Lückes, and her nursing staff did he receive unflinching courtesy and consideration, but even here there was a sense of a certain instinctive constraint. They were, he recognized, but nurses carrying out a necessary duty in a professional way.

While Joseph now had rooms of his own, the burden of nursing him remained no light matter; and in spite of the care lavished on him, his day-to-day life was far from easy. His condition continued to become more troublesome; his hip was painful, his movements slow and stubborn. The weight of his enlarged limbs tired him quickly, and he found it impossible to perform many small tasks on his own account. Even in bed it was difficult for him to rest since he found it impossible to lie flat. Should he do so, the weight of the fleshy and bony growths on his skull made it unmanageable and he was overcome by a sensation of the head rolling backwards, stretching and constricting the neck muscles. To sleep, he found it essential to crouch upright on the bed in a foetal parody, his legs drawn up, his arms clasped about them and his great head resting on his knees.

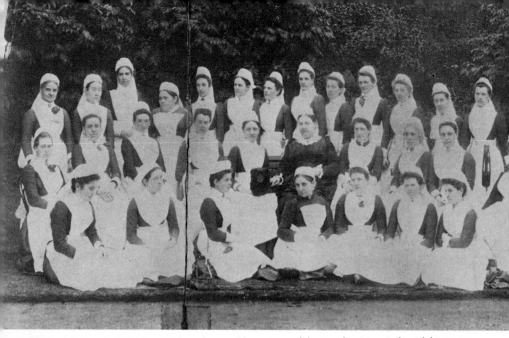

Plate 46. Miss Eva Lückes, the notable matron of the London Hospital, with her team of nursing sisters in 1892

Plate 47. One of the wards at the London Hospital illustrated in the *Illustrated London News*, 21 July 1888

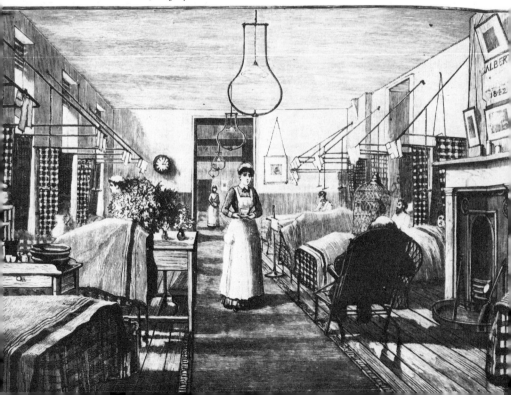

There were occasions when Treves found himself peering in on something of the boredom and loneliness to which Joseph was essentially condemned all his life. There were periods when Joseph became hopelessly despondent. For hours at a time, when he thought himself unobserved, he might sit staring before him, beating slowly and rhythmically on his pillow or the arm of his chair with his deformed right arm. It seemed to Treves that Joseph was keeping time to a tune heard only in his mind – one which he was unable to voice, for he could never attempt to whistle or even sing. The surgeon saw the habit as an expression of inward cheerfulness, but a doctor today might rather interpret it as a classic depressive symptom.

Once, during such a period of depression, Joseph startled Treves by returning to the subject of his future care. It was clear that he still had not grasped that his new quarters were his to occupy for life. Some of the suggestions which members of the public made when Carr Gomm launched the appeal found an echo in his own thoughts, for he inquired about the time when he would have to move on once again, suggesting that he might perhaps find a refuge in some out-of-the-way spot, such as a lighthouse or in an asylum for the blind. It was a distressing task trying to convince this small and infinitely vulnerable man that he had no need to journey further.

But Treves was also coming to realize that Joseph's sanctuary in the basement rooms was in danger of turning into a prison. Joseph's sense of isolation was increasing and Treves felt certain that much of his patient's distress sprang from the loneliness life had forced upon him. To Treves it seemed that these sufferings came at least in part from having been rejected by so many fellow human beings. More than anything else, he felt it necessary to convince Joseph that he could be accepted on equal terms as a normal person. One possible solution might be to introduce him to people who would disregard his hideous appearance and communicate with him with courtesy and consideration. For this particular task, who could be more suitable than a well-bred lady of the British upper middle class, versed in composure and social virtue? Treves cast about in his mind for such a person who might be persuaded to meet Merrick and who could be relied upon to be strong-minded enough to keep her nerve whatever her inner feelings, for the failure of such an experiment might well turn into an irreparable disaster.

At last, Treves said, he asked a friend, 'a young and pretty widow, if she thought she could enter Merrick's room with a smile, wish him good morning and shake him by the hand'. It was essential that she should betray no trace of revulsion or embarrassment. The young widow whom Treves approached was Mrs Leila Maturin, whose husband, Dr Leslie Maturin, had died in 1883 within only two months of their marriage. She listened to Treves's proposal and his description of the Elephant Man, and without hesitation accepted the role in which he was casting her: an introduction of beauty to the beast, though with strict limits on the hopes of a transformation.

Treves accompanied Leila Maturin as she was taken to the little basement room to meet Joseph. She entered his room with an easy grace, smiling as she approached him, reaching out and taking his hand as Treves presented him to her.

It was all too much. Joseph could not speak. Slowly he released her hand and slowly he bent his great head forward to his knees as he broke into heart-rending sobs and wept uncontrollably. The meeting ended as quickly as it had begun.

Afterwards Joseph confided to a rather shaken Treves that this was the first time any strange woman had smiled at him, let alone taken his hand in greeting. The event itself was, however, a landmark, ushering in a wholly new phase in the life of the Elephant Man. Treves pinpointed it as a moment when a renewal of self-confidence began for Joseph Merrick. The old hurts and haunting fears of spying eyes and whispered wonderings slowly began to heal and dissolve. The impulse to hide himself away from the world was changed into a renewed curiosity and a wish to reach out to grasp some of the small everyday experiences which were commonplace in the lives of ordinary people but hitherto as beyond Joseph's reach as if they were something to do with life on the moon itself.

After this time Treves had the impression that Joseph fell in love with every attractive woman he met – though 'in a humble and devotional way', he was careful to add. Treves's thoroughness in ensuring that no mirror came his way in which he might catch a chance glimpse of himself meanwhile began to lead Joseph to forget the full horror of his appearance. 'He was amorous,' said Treves. 'He would like to have been a lover, to have walked with the beloved object in the languorous shades of some beautiful garden and to have poured into her ear all the glowing utterances that he had rehearsed in his heart.' Treves sensed that behind Merrick's musings about finding a refuge in an asylum for the blind was the idea that he might be able to raise a spark of affection in the heart of some blind girl who could not see the disfigurement of his flesh.

Such thoughts were clearly safer left sublimated in the realms of romantic chivalry. Treves was a directly robust character among Victorian doctors, a scientific realist as well as a man of imagination. The sharp irony of the fact that Joseph's genitalia remained perfectly normal among all his deformities cannot have been beyond him.

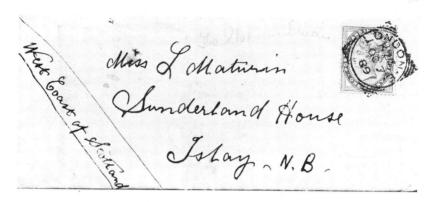

Plates 48a–b. The letter of thanks and its envelope which Joseph Merrick wrote to Mrs Maturin and which is the only known surviving item of his correspondence

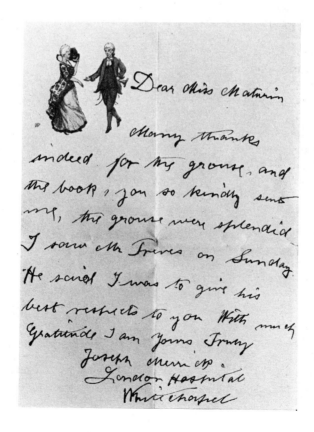

CHAPTER 9

'Such a Gentle, Kindly Man, Poor Thing!'

Even during the early days following his admission to the London Hospital, the case of Joseph Merrick began to attract the attention of people who were in a position to bring their social influence to focus on his behalf. Outstanding among these was the actress, Mrs Kendal, to whose actor husband, W.H. Kendal, Mr Wardell Cardew mentioned the fact of Joseph Merrick having been in Ostend. Wardell Cardew then went on to suggest that Mr Kendal might care to go to the London Hospital to see the Elephant Man for himself, and he did so. In fact Kendal had studied medicine for a time before deciding to make his career in the theatre, and among his friends was John Bland-Sutton. He had continued to keep up his interest in medical topics.

When he returned home from his visit, his wife asked him whether he had enjoyed himself amid all the medical activity. According to her memoirs, *Dame Madge Kendal by Herself*, he replied decisively:

'No ... I have not. I have seen the most fearful sight of my life.'
'Don't tell me about it,' I replied.
'The extraordinary thing,' declared my husband, 'is that out of the distorted frame came the most musical voice.'

The experience so affected him that he could hardly speak. When he recovered, he told me that Mr Cardew had said they would never allow Merrick to be in the hospital permanently, although he ought to be in there, as it was not fit that he should be seen in public.

'Wouldn't they let him remain in the hospital,' I asked, 'if the money was raised to pay for his keep?'

At this time Madge Kendal was appearing at the St James's Theatre,

Piccadilly, with her husband's business partner in theatrical management, Mr John Hare, in *The Hobby Horse*, a new play by the rising young playwright Arthur Pinero. The excellent cast also included Mrs Beerbohm Tree, and the drama critic of *Punch* said he really did not care in what Mrs Kendal and Mr Hare appeared, their playing was so excellent. Evidently the play was not vintage Pinero, but Mrs Kendal had the rewarding and appropriate part of an irreproachable married woman whose one peculiarity was her philanthropic hobby of turning the family house into a refuge for waifs and strays, to her husband's great exasperation. Yet it was a success with the theatre-going public, for whom Mrs Kendal was a star performer who could do no wrong.

Plate 49. Madge Kendal performs the leading role in Pinero's play, *The Hobby Horse*

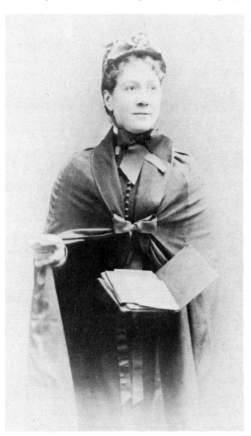

Madge Kendal had been born into a family with strong theatrical antece-
dents, the Robertsons, and among her ancestors was James Robertson, an
actor and playwright who was a contemporary of David Garrick well known
in the fashionable centres of Bath and York. Several generations of theatrical
managers followed, and one of her elder brothers (there were twenty-two
children in the family) was T.W. Robertson, the dramatist who had a
decisive influence in introducing the new realism on to the Victorian stage.
He saw this as a principle which would affect a production as a whole, from
the playscript to the style of the acting and the production details, and he
was one of the first to stipulate that when he asked for coat-pegs in the
scenery they should be real coat-pegs on which real coats could be hung, not
mere painted simulations.

When Madge Robertson married W.H. Kendal in 1869, her career as an
accomplished and popular actress was already firmly launched. Her husband
was similarly becoming well known as an actor manager, though in the end
it was his wife's fame which was the more durable. Nevertheless, their
partnership lasted throughout their lives and they became a byword for
respectable example in the theatrical world where a general raffishness set as
ever the more usual tone.

In all her life Madge Kendal never flinched from performing acts of charity.
Many years after the events which concerned the Elephant Man, she was to
claim that she had been the one responsible for anonymously launching the
fund which brought Merrick the financial security to maintain him in the
London Hospital. Be that as it may, it has to be emphasized that while her
husband met Merrick, she herself probably never did so. The chapter on
'The Elephant Man' in her published memoirs contains no indication of a
personal encounter. The tone is detached and she relies on Treves's already
published description to sketch in his appearance. Her incessantly crowded
career must, in any case, have left her little enough time for charitable visits
in the manner of ladies of greater leisure.

Nevertheless she represented the starting point to a network of personages
who would mobilize sympathy for Joseph Merrick's welfare and incidentally
enrich his experience of a social life in the few years which remained to him.
In the meantime, he had begun to explore within the limits of the exploration
he could manage: a few limping steps in the darkness of late evening, a
shuffling from his room, a painful toiling up the concrete steps and then the
cold stillness of Bedstead Square with its shadows, the far-away glow of the
high ward windows and the occasional echo of distant footsteps. Yet it
evoked in him a sense of freedom to stand unmolested in the open air. With
each nocturnal excursion, his confidence increased until at last he was able

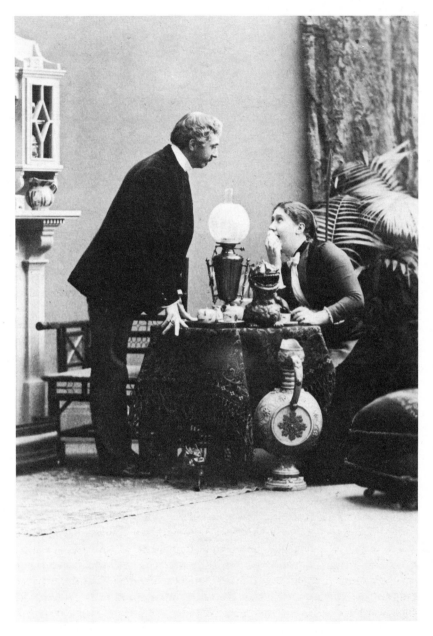

Plate 50. Mr and Mrs Kendal act together in a play called *A Scrap of Paper*

to make his way from the square, skirting beyond the patches of light thrown from windows, picking his way through the rubble of builders' materials that littered the ground where new extensions were being built, moving in a hesitant exploration round beyond the end of the great block of the East Wing until he came to the hospital gardens and walked alone in the darkness, feeling the grass soft beneath his feet, savouring the forgotten scent of night flowers.

In the daytime, he spied cautiously upon the comings and goings in Bedstead Square. He had learnt to recognize the faces of those who passed daily above his window, and the workmen in their turn became aware of the unseen but watchful presence behind the curtains in the little basement room. Here, too, he unexpectedly found friends. Mr Taylor, the chief engineer, came one day to introduce Charles Taylor, his youngest son, a lad about seventeen years old. A friendship quickly sprang up between them, and after that the youth came regularly, bringing his violin to play in private recital for Joseph's entertainment.

Mrs Kendal sent him gifts, the first being an early gramophone of the type invented by Edison only about ten years before, the recordings for which were made on cylinders rotated by a hand-worked handle at the side. Joseph wrote to thank Mrs Kendal for her kindness, and in fact he wrote her letters on at least several occasions. Alas, the letters did not survive. She presented them to the London Hospital, but they could no longer be traced when she came to write her memoirs in the early 1930s. He also sent her one of the cardboard models he had constructed with the aid of the nurses. It was a delicately detailed model of a Gothic church, and this has survived, being preserved today in the museum of the London Hospital Medical College.

In one of his letters to Mrs Kendal, Joseph mentioned that he hoped one day to be able to learn basket-work. She promptly arranged for an instructor to teach him the craft. Now his room became littered with bundles of cane and small basket-work articles waiting to be given to whoever would accept them. The first basket that he completed he sent to Mrs Kendal herself.

Since it was evidently not possible for her to go to see him, Joseph requested that she might send him some photographs. These she forwarded, and he displayed them triumphantly in his room.

It came as rather a surprise to Treves to find how Joseph was developing into something of a celebrity. The letter to *The Times* had had the effect of arousing not only a phenomenal charitable response but also a widespread curiosity. Requests to visit the Elephant Man were being received by the hospital. Within a few months of the disturbing incident of his meeting with the pretty young widow, Treves was reaching the rueful conclusion that

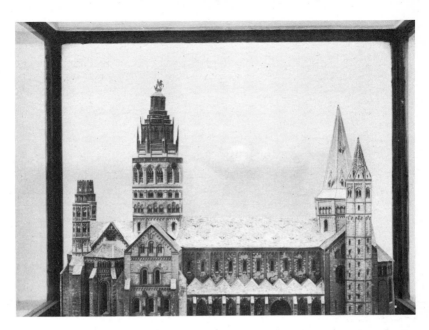

Plate 51. The cardboard model of the church which Merrick constructed for Mrs Kendal

every lady of note in the social sphere would soon be making the journey to the hospital to be escorted to the basement rooms and introduced. Each one who came was forewarned about his appearance, and each one sturdily summoned the courage to greet him with a smile and handshake, and even to spend a few minutes in conversation.

To begin with, Joseph was reticent towards his guests, but every introduction seemed to bring him a little more confidence, and each day his manner became more self-assured. Treves was still having to act as interpreter. Joseph's speech was improving with practice but it remained indistinct. His visitors, though perhaps drawn mainly by curiosity or the fact that it was fast becoming the fashionable thing to visit Joseph Merrick, were entirely benevolent. They brought him gifts, so that his rooms grew bright with ornaments and pictures. Sometimes he received autographed portraits or photographs of the ladies who called, and these joined the others displayed about the room. Some of the gentlemen left money to be spent on his behalf, and in this Treves acted as steward. The gifts which pleased Joseph most, however, were books, for he was slowly accumulating quite a respectable library and his spare time was increasingly given over to reading.

The paradox was not lost on Treves, as he saw Joseph emerging into this object of patronage and interest. His protégé, once a homeless waif shunned by virtually all who encountered him, was beginning to become the sought-after acquaintance of duchesses and countesses. It is doubtful, however, whether the surgeon could have taken the irony the one step further, and have seen the accident of his own intervention as carrying Joseph's career as a freak on to a new, unimaginable level of success; or himself as the *alter ego* to Mr Tom Norman, the showman whom he despised so consistently.

As Joseph lost the last of his reticence, he would speak relaxedly and strike up acquaintanceships with anyone who paused to acknowledge his presence. It became his habit to sit at his window so he could have a word with whoever happened to pass in Bedstead Square. He no longer hung back behind the curtains, and regular passers-by would often stop and call to inspect his more recent gifts or to hear tales of the distinguished guests he had entertained. They were tales told with an innocent jubilation, steeped more in wonder than in pride. On a few occasions he wandered away from his room in search of company, and once he raised an alarm by appearing without warning at the entrance to one of the main wards. Only a flurry of nurses rushing to gather about him and shepherd him back to his own quarters prevented his sudden presence from delivering a shock to the other patients.

Joseph's fresh curiosity about the outside world naturally extended to Treves. He questioned the surgeon shyly about himself and the home he lived in with his family. He seemed particularly inquisitive about the house itself, asking wistfully about its arrangement and how it looked. At last he remarked obliquely that he should like to see the inside of a 'real' house. The simple artisan terrace dwellings, such as he knew in Leicester, or the lodgings of the freakshow circuit, could clearly never have counted as such. It was the elegant town houses of the rich, which he glimpsed standing splendid and remote during his travels, their doors perpetually closed to him, which teased his imagination. With the help of his reading, he had been able to people and furnish their splendid interiors, but now he wanted to measure his imagined images against the facts.

Treves recognized the wish that was implied by Joseph's mentioning the subject. Within a few days he arranged for him to be taken to his own house at 6 Wimpole Street, safely hidden inside a hansom cab. It may be assumed that the household was suitably prepared: that Treves's daughters, Enid, aged eight, and Hetty, aged four, were safely out of the way when Joseph was hurried across the pavements and into the hall's seclusion.

Solemnly Treves escorted his guest from room to room. It turned out to be a slow process, for Joseph would pause to examine every object, gazing at each piece of furniture, each curtain, each fabric with almost comically exaggerated interest. As they progressed, Treves became aware of a sense of unease within himself. The house seemed to be in some way falling short of Joseph's expectations. He had clearly expected to find a larger and grander establishment and was puzzled by the lack of liveried footmen and other servants in constant attendance. (Treves himself, when writing of his consulting room, once described it as the smallest in London, 'not much more than a cupboard with a fireplace and window'.)

Anxious that Joseph should not be disappointed, while hoping to explain circumstances and perhaps retrieve a certain lost prestige, Treves explained that this was never meant to be the home of an aristocrat, but was rather a town house, built in the more modest style of dwellings as described in the novels of Jane Austen. Joseph, who had read *Emma*, accepted the comparison with a polite gravity.

From the time of its foundation in the eighteenth century, the London Hospital was forced to wage a continuous battle against not only lack of funds but also a shortage of accommodation. In 1887 two sets of new buildings were nearing completion. On the south side of Bedstead Square, beyond the end of the East Wing, the new Nurses Home was being constructed. In Turner Street, at the side of the hospital, new accommodation for the Medical College was almost finished. By the spring of 1887, both buildings were completed, and on 21 May the official ceremony was held to declare them open.

The Prince and Princess of Wales accepted the invitation to perform the ceremony, and their carriage arrived at the main gates at five o'clock in the afternoon on a day wet with a steady drizzle. They were received by a formal reception party headed by the president of the London Hospital, George William, second Duke of Cambridge, Commander in Chief of the Army and a cousin of Queen Victoria's.

As a young man of twenty-one, George William had defied the conventions expected of a royal duke by marrying a commoner who was also an actress. His successful life-long marriage was quietly ignored by the monarch, the court and society at large. He had been on active service during the Crimean War, and had had his horse shot from under him at the battle of Inkerman, though he then managed to rally a hundred survivors from the division to break through the encircling Russians. By the 1880s the old warrior was ageing and gruffly formidable. He had as good as inherited the presidency of the hospital from his father, who died in 1850, and was untiring in the

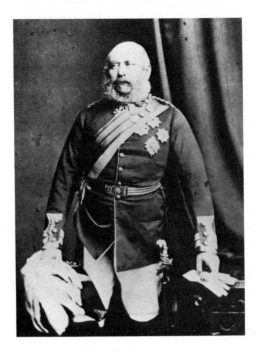

Plate 52. H.R.H. George William, second Duke of Cambridge

support he gave and rallied. He graced official occasions, spoke at innumerable dinners, presided over charitable gatherings and maintained a determined supervision over the hospital's variegated activities. He never hesitated to voice displeasure should someone omit to consult him over any important piece of institutional business, though his irascibility was in general recognized as concealing genuine concern and kindness. He had even continued to meet these commitments during the years of Queen Victoria's retirement from public life after the death of the Prince Consort in 1861, when he shouldered many of the public tasks expected from the head of state.

The Prince and Princess of Wales themselves kept up an association with the London Hospital from 1864 onwards. One of their joint duties in that year, which followed the year of their marriage, had been to lay the foundation stone for the new block known as the Alexandra Wing. For 21 May 1887, the plans were more elaborate. The royal party would first be conducted to the new Nurses Home, to be received in the dining-room by the matron, Miss Eva Lückes, at the head of her nursing staff. The chapel choir would then sing a hymn, the suffragan Bishop of Bedford would read a collect and the Duke of Cambridge would ask the Princess of Wales to declare the building, to be called the Alexandra Home, open. From there the party would be escorted to the new Medical College buildings, where further speeches would be delivered and a similar ceremony performed by the Prince of Wales; but on the way the royal dignitaries would be invited to visit several wards.

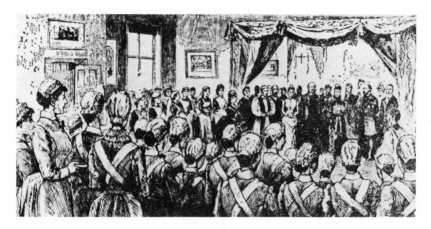

Plate 53. The Princess of Wales declares the new Nurses Home open at the London Hospital on 21 May 1887 in an illustration from the *Illustrated London News*

The slow, dignified procession duly passed from bed to bed, though the princess was visibly moved by the spectacle of so much suffering. Then, from the wards, the party descended to the basements of the East Wing so that the princess might be introduced to the Elephant Man, who had by that time been in the hospital almost a year. She was warned that his appearance was literally shocking, and Frederick Treves accompanied the party as a matter of course.

Thus Joseph Merrick suddenly found his small room flooded with strangers, but the most important person among them was for him the Princess of Wales. She had entered the room with a relaxed grace, smiled and taken the introduction with perfect serenity, shaking him by the hand and sitting beside his chair so that she might talk to him. She examined his curios and gifts with an interest that left him transported with wonder. The Prince of Wales also spoke to him, being quietly amused to spot Mrs Kendal among the collection of autographed portraits. And then, as suddenly as it appeared, the royal party withdrew, leaving Joseph overwhelmed with excitement.

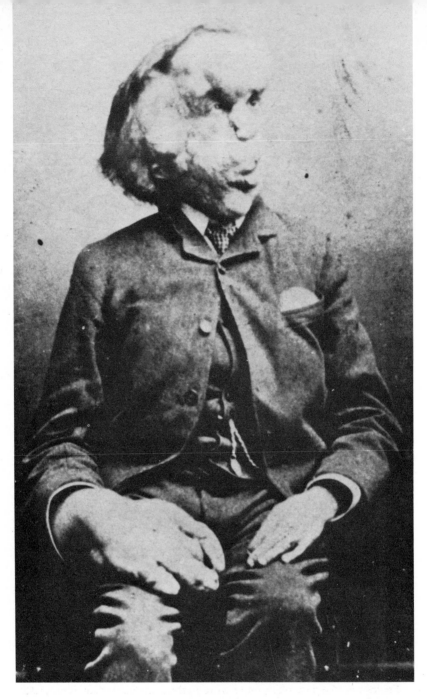

Plate 54. Joseph Merrick, dressed for a portrait photograph in his 'Sunday best'

Later that night, the Duke of Cambridge confided to his diary some details of the afternoon:

> 1887, May 21st – Went to the London Hospital, where as President I received at 5 o'clock the Prince and Princess of Wales, who came to open the new home just finished for the Nurses of the Hospital. We passed through the wards, saw the unfortunate man called the elephant man, who is a painful sight to look at, though intelligent in himself, and then I read an address to the Prince and Princess to which the Prince replied. It was very wet, but we were able to return in open carriages. The crowds in the streets were very enthusiastic. All went off well.

It was probably on this occasion, though he did not mention it, that the Duke of Cambridge discreetly presented Joseph with a silver watch.

The following afternoon he paid a call on his mother, the aged Duchess of Cambridge. Lady Geraldine Somerset, who attended the duchess, kept a journal for her, and in this she recorded the duke's visit:

> May 22nd, 1887
> ... At 3 came the Duke. He gave H.R.H. an account ... of the Princess of Wales ... at the London Hospital, tearing up her bouquet, to give a flower of it to each sick child & each sick woman. Of their having seen the Elephant-man, poor creature – a sad spectacle! *enormous*, with two great bosses on the forehead really like an elephant's head, & a protruding face like a snout, one *enormous* hand like the foot of an elephant, the other, the left hand, extraordinarily, exceptionally *small*! He can never go out, he is mobbed so, & lives therefore a prisoner; he is less disgusting to see than might be, because he is such a gentle, kindly man, poor thing! ...

The Duke of Cambridge had clearly put across a graphic account of Joseph to his mother. On his own side Joseph treasured the memory of the meeting, recounting the events over and over, though the excitement was not yet finished with. In due course he received a small package from Marlborough House. It contained a signed photograph of the Princess of Wales, sent so that he might include it in his collection. For Joseph, whose emotions lay constantly only just below the surface, the gift was overwhelming, and he broke down and wept over it. It was so important to him that he could scarcely bear for even Treves to touch it. It was framed for him, and he hung it in his room, treating it as almost a sacred object.

Treves suggested that he should write to the princess to thank her, and he did so, naïvely beginning his letter, 'My dear Princess' and signing it off,

'Yours very sincerely'. When asked by Joseph to read the letter to see if it was all right, Treves was so touched by it that he let it go as it stood. The princess visited Joseph again on other occasions, and when Christmas came sent him not one but three Christmas cards, each one personally inscribed with a message on the back. A further effect of her interest was to amplify the volume of his other illustrious visitors. 'It became a cult among the personal friends of the Princess,' wrote John Bland-Sutton, 'to visit the Elephant Man in the London Hospital.' Neither did the Prince of Wales forget him. From time to time a bag of game would arrive for Joseph's table following a shoot on the royal estates.

Some years later, at a charity garden fête given by Sir William Treloar in Chelsea, Mrs Kendal was selling autographed photographs of herself on one of the stalls. The former Prince of Wales, by now King Edward VII, surveyed each picture in turn before solemnly informing her, 'I think, Mrs Kendal, you must have given your best photographs to James Merrick.' Evidently something that King Edward and Frederick Treves had in common was a degree of difficulty with the Elephant Man's correct Christian name.

Christmas at the London Hospital was always a thoroughly observed festival. For weeks beforehand the nursing staff would prepare decorations for the wards; for days gifts would pour in at the main gates. Festivities would begin quietly in the early hours of Christmas morning when a choir of sisters and nurses moved from ward to ward, singing carols. Then, during the morning, Father Christmas himself would arrive, helped by an assorted band of fairies to distribute a present to every patient in the hospital.

At midday, as the resident doctors carved the turkeys in the lobbies to each of their wards, the patients settled down to a special dinner sanctioned by the house committee. It always finished with a slice of plum pudding. For the sisters, nurses and probationers, there were special dinners enriched with delicacies provided by the senior surgeons and physicians. In the afternoon, the consultant staff came down with their children to see the shows, for the residents, nurses, students and dentals then dressed up to tour the hospital and perform amateur entertainments for the patients. For the children, there was a Punch and Judy show. In the evening, as the wards settled into darkness, a Christmas dance was given for the wardmaids, and later on there was a midnight supper for the scrubbers.

The coming of Christmas for Joseph Merrick meant in the first place the arrival of his Christmas cards, not only the polite cards from nurses and staff, but those from the various visitors who had befriended him, including

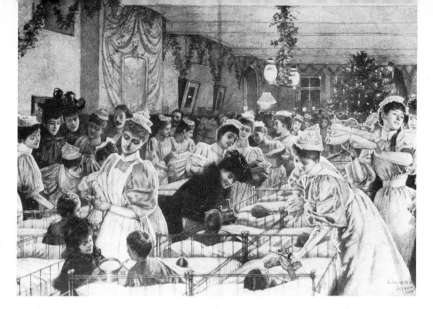

Plate 55. Christmas at the London Hospital. An illustration from the *Graphic*, 25 December 1897

those which always came from Princess Alexandra. There were also many personal gifts.

One year, shortly before Christmas, Treves asked Joseph what he felt he would like, for several gifts of money had been handed in to be spent for his benefit. Joseph showed no hesitation. He had seen an advertisement for a gentleman's dressing case with silver fittings which appealed to him so much that he had kept the cutting from the newspaper. The set consisted of silver-backed hairbrushes and comb, a silver shoehorn and a hat brush as well as ivory-handled razors and toothbrushes. It seemed an incongruous choice, but Treves understood the feelings behind it and purchased the set at once. He intervened only to prepare the gift by removing the mirror and carefully filling the cigarette case with cigarettes, though he knew that Joseph never smoked and never could with his deformed lips; but then every item in the case was equally useless to him in a utilitarian sense.

The dressing case turned out to be a perfect prop for Joseph's imagination. In the privacy of his small room, sitting quietly as he arranged its contents, opening and closing the cigarette case, he became an elegant, sophisticated man-about-town, preparing in his dressing-room for some formal dinner or glittering occasion.

By this stage Treves was beginning to take a positive relish in introducing Joseph to new experiences. There was about it, he found, something of the pleasure to be derived from watching a child's astonishment when it encounters a new and unexpected wonder. Among Joseph's unfulfilled social aspirations was being able to have an evening out at a West End theatre, but the difficulties here were immense. Should any audience catch a glimpse of Joseph Merrick among them, it could hardly be expected to pay much further attention to anything going forward on the stage. The matter, however, was carried to the ears of Mrs Kendal, who saw at once that one answer could be for Joseph to watch the stage from a position of concealment. She moved to exploit her social contacts, and went to call on the Baroness Burdett-Coutts.

The baroness, who kept a private box in the Theatre Royal, Drury Lane, was one of the richest women in nineteenth-century England. She was a notable philanthropist, and a patroness of the arts and of the theatre in particular, who had set up Henry Irving for his famous period of occupancy at the Lyceum Theatre. By now in her seventies, she still held a controlling interest in Coutts, the bankers founded by her grandfather, and so was banker to the royal family. Both the first Duke and Duchess of Cambridge were her friends, as was the second duke, the president of the London Hospital. Guests as diverse as the Duke of Wellington, Sir Robert Peel, Samuel Wilberforce, W.E. Gladstone and Benjamin Disraeli had sat at her dinner table.

She was formidably well informed, cultivating, as well as politicians, scientists such as Michael Faraday and Joseph Hooker, or writers such as Charles Dickens, who dedicated *Martin Chuzzlewit* to her. She helped to finance the expeditions to Africa of David Livingstone, and later those of Henry Morton Stanley. Her vast fortune was used for prodigious acts of charity, in which, while he was alive, Charles Dickens would advise her.

The baroness had made her private box at Drury Lane available to many people in the past, including Dickens and his family, but the prospect of the Elephant Man occupying it caused her some anxieties. What, she asked, would the consequences be if an unfortunate woman should unexpectedly catch sight of him; what dreadful effect might it not have? Mrs Kendal assured Baroness Burdett-Coutts that arrangements would be in the responsible hands of Frederick Treves, that no one would see the Elephant Man arriving, or leaving the theatre, and that steps would be taken to ensure he was in no way visible to the audience. The baroness withdrew her objections and the operation was planned.

It was by now the pantomime season at Drury Lane, the Christmas pantomime, of course, being a firmly established tradition in the Victorian theatre. The famous sequence of annual pantomimes at Drury Lane which Augustus Harris mounted there after he took over its management in 1880 had become bywords for rich and elaborate spectacle and the use of star names from the London music halls to play the leads. As *The Times* critic remarked in 1883:

On the stage commanded by Augustus Harris the tales of Fairyland are annually illustrated with a magnificence which sets criticism at nought. They hardly fall within the domain of drama. They are a dream, a phantasmagoria, the baseless fabric of a vision, and are best appreciated in a spirit of child-like wonderment.

Unfortunately, neither Treves nor Madge Kendal tell us which of those famous productions it was planned that Joseph should see, but the year in which Joseph Merrick was taken to Drury Lane, with Madge Kendal's help, was almost certainly 1887. It could hardly have been the year before, since the business of Joseph's admission to the London Hospital was at that time only just being resolved. From the summer of 1888, the movements and preoccupations of the Kendals make it extremely unlikely that Mrs Kendal would have been available in London to assist in the adventure. On 21 July 1888, the long partnership between the Kendals and Mr John Hare at the St James's Theatre finally broke. With *The Weaker Sex*, a new play by Arthur Pinero, under their wings, the Kendals established a company of their own. There were problems to be ironed out in the play's presentation, and at the outset they took it on a tour of the provinces.

The first night was at Manchester on 28 September 1888. Not until six months later did they bring the production to London, opening at the Court Theatre on 16 March 1889. They stayed at the Court Theatre throughout the summer, planning their first great tour of the United States. By the autumn they had left England, opening triumphantly at the Fifth Avenue Theatre, New York, in October 1889. They did not return to England until 26 June 1890.

Had Joseph seen the pantomime for 1888, he would have witnessed the début in pantomime of the great comedian Dan Leno, in *The Babes in the Wood*. As it was, it seems that the one he saw must have been *Puss in Boots*, and the pamphlet *The Elephant Man*, published in 1888 and reproduced as Appendix Two (see page 227), gives further confirmation. It is doubtful if he would have been appreciative of Dan Leno in any case, since the element of the comedians did not hold much appeal for him.

The book for the 1887 production of *Puss in Boots* was written by E.L. Blanchard, who wrote every pantomime at Drury Lane between 1852 and 1888, and had been responsible in his day for giving the *genre* a certain literary quality. Each year under Augustus Harris's management, however,

Mr Blanchard complained ever more bitterly at the way his scripts were reworked ruthlessly to make room for some ambitious scenic procession or the comic business of the music-hall artists. The tradition was changing and Blanchard could only grouse as he once did in his diary: '. . . hardly anything done as I intended it, or spoken as I had written: the music-hall element is crushing out the rest and the good old fairy-tales never again to be illustrated as they should be.' In fact Harris was giving the public of the 1880s what it wanted, and his pantomimes usually justified the lavish financial investments which went into mounting them.

Not that any such considerations were even of academic interest to Joseph, for whom the whole affair was to turn out to be an experience of unexampled wonder from the moment when he was smuggled into Drury Lane Theatre from a carriage with drawn blinds. Permission had been given to use the royal entrance with its private staircase. 'All went well,' said Treves, 'and no one saw a figure, more monstrous than any on the stage, mount the staircase or cross the corridor.' Once in the private box, a trio of ward sisters, wearing normal evening dress, had volunteered to sit in the front row to create a shield. Treves then sat with Joseph, effectively concealed in the shadows at the back of the box.

Plate 56. The deeply recessed boxes at Drury Lane Theatre as they were in the auditorium in 1887. The one Joseph Merrick occupied was probably that nearest the stage

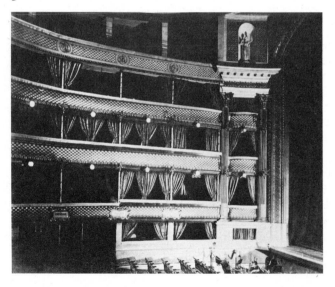

To imagine what Joseph felt at this moment it would be necessary to have total recall of the biggest treat of one's childhood, before the encroachment of experience made such an absorption of innocent and uncritical vision impossible. Under the direction of Mr Jimmy Glover, the resident conductor, the theatre band struck up the overture, and then the curtain rose on the opening scene. Mr Blanchard took his story line from the fairy-tale which Charles Perrault made familiar to generations of children by including it in his collection of nursery tales in the seventeenth century, though it had considerably more ancient origins in Italian folk story.

The youngest son of a miller, when his father dies, inherits nothing but the cat. So he sets out in company with his feline friend to seek his fortune in the world. One day, while he is swimming, a royal coach approaches, and the quick-witted cat cries out to it to stop, for, it says, his master is drowning. Dragged from the water, the bewildered youth finds himself being introduced by the cat to the King, Queen and Princess as the Marquis of Carabas. After this incident the boy and his cat travel on to an ogre's castle, where the cat tricks the monster into turning himself, first, into a lion, then into a mouse; whereupon he falls on him and eats him up. In this way, having taken possession of the ogre's castle, lands and treasure, the cat is able to present them to his master and so make him a fit match for the princess of the realm. Naturally, the young couple have already fallen in love the moment their eyes engaged.

For Augustus Harris, the simple scaffolding of the traditional tale provided a springboard for a variety of extravagances, not all of which had much to do with advancing the story. The list of performers was long, for there were the music-hall songs, the balletic interludes, the harlequinade and the climax of the transformation scene all to be incorporated. The part of Jocelyn, the miller's son, otherwise known as the Marquis of Carabas, was taken by Miss Tilly Wadman as principal boy, 'handsome and plays and sings charmingly', according to *Punch*, though *The Times* felt her singing 'was not always very true, but she makes a capital Burlesque Prince'. Master Charles Lauri took the part of Puss, and Letty Lind, a rising star among the dancing girls of the Gaiety Theatre who had made her début there only that year, was the Princess Sweetheart.

'Neatly tripping, lightly dancing Letty Lind,' enthused *The Times*, 'who has already made herself a favourite with the children and their attendants.' 'These are leggy days,' said *Punch* more cryptically.

The part of the King was taken by Herbert Campbell, a comic singer from the music halls who came to specialize in dame parts, though not on this occasion. The Queen was played by Harry Nicholls, a light comedy actor.

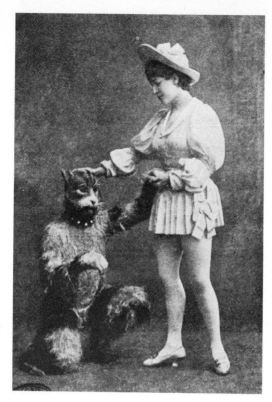

Plate 57. Charles Lauri as Puss and Tilly Wadman as principal boy in the 1887 pantomime

The one [said *The Times*] is a pantomime monarch worthy of Thackeray in *The Rose and the Ring*, and the other a depressed but loquacious Queen who manages to get in more than one word edgeways. All the matrimonial squabbles, all the domestic wrangling, all the polite sarcasms and family jars are conceived in the best spirit of humour by two actors who are singularly observant ... The fun they get out of the journey in the stage coach, the incident of the pretended drowning of the Marquis of Carabas, and the struggle for supremacy with the costermonger's donkey, are all in the best and most legitimate spirit of pantomime fun.

The harlequinade which featured towards the end was, of course, a link back to the very origins of pantomime burlesque, and by now almost an anachronism in the changing tradition. The leading part of the clown was in this case taken by Mr Harry Payne, who was resident clown in the Drury Lane pantomimes from 1883 until 1894, the year before his death. Prior to

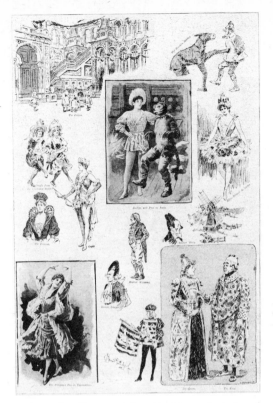

Plate 58. A page from the *Illustrated London News* depicting the *Puss in Boots* pantomime

this he used to play Harlequin, and his father, W.H. Payne, had as a pantomimist worked with the great Grimaldi himself.

But, said Treves, Merrick 'did not like the ogres and the giants, while the funny men impressed him as irreverent. Having no experience as a boy of romping and ragging, or practical jokes and "larks", he had little sympathy with the doings of the clown ...' On the other hand, he did react with pleasure when the policeman's dignity was decisively undermined by his being smacked about the face and knocked backwards. Whatever he may once have witnessed of police officiousness towards the freakshows must have been a factor in his response in this instance. For the rest, it was the spectacle which entranced him.

His reaction was not so much that of delight as of wonder and amazement. He was awed. He was enthralled. The spectacle left him

Plate 59 (overleaf). The spectacular court scene from *Puss in Boots*

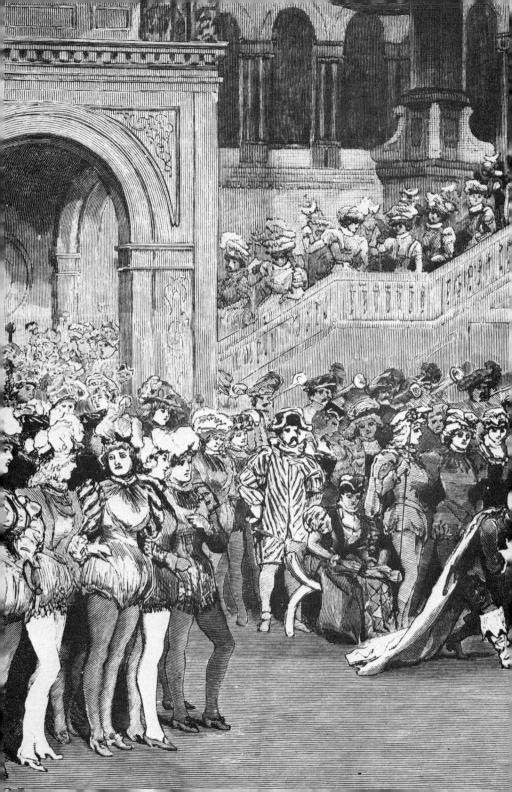

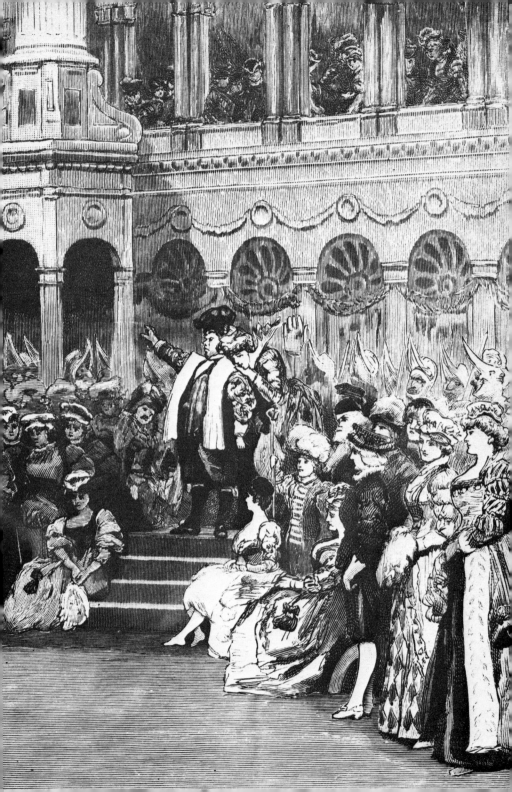

speechless, so that if he were spoken to he took no heed. He often seemed to be panting for breath . . . [he was] thrilled by a vision that was almost beyond his comprehension . . . The splendour and display impressed him, but, I think, the ladies of the ballet took a still greater hold on his fancy.

There were three 'Spectacular Scenes' which punctuated Augustus Harris's ambitious production. Two of them, according to *The Times*, 'were veritable dreams of beauty', the first showing the inner court of the King and Queen's palace: '. . . a dazzling structure of marble, with high raised galleries, lofty columns and a grand staircase down which a dozen people can walk abreast'. And down the staircase tripped chambermaids in yellow and blue gowns, to be followed by a procession, heralded by trumpeters, of the entire court in costumes which exhausted 'the whole catalogue of colours'. The *Illustrated London News* was so carried away as to exclaim that there were 'bits of this stage production worthy of Paolo Veronese'.

The second great spectacle came once the pantomime cat had cunningly disposed of the ogre. The vast hall of the ogre's castle was suddenly seen to be 'filled with warriors in complete armour', some mounted but others on foot. These forces launched themselves into an elaborate drill routine with their halberds, and then a great expanse of tapestry at the back was drawn aside to reveal yet another staircase, down which there swarmed

> . . . some countless warriors in gold and silver armour followed by knights accompanied by their squires and standard bearers. The entire stage in its length and breadth is filled with glittering metal, nodding plumes and fluttering pennons which rival in colour the whole tribe of butterflies.

The third and last spectacle was the one against which the fairy ballet took place and which became the transformation scene. In the foreground was an oak glade, the boughs of the mighty trees overarching the stage and their trunks surrounded by a rich array of fern and foxglove. Beyond the glade stretched a lake, golden in summer light and surrounded by more trees, while a line of distant hills on the backcloth closed the enchanted vista. The object of it all, said the *Illustrated London News*, was

> . . . to present, by means of children and girls, a wedding bouquet. It is charmingly and fancifully carried out, and the most delightful result of white flowers and green leaves, maidenhair fern, roses, lilies, stephan-otis, daisies and azalea is attained at minimum cost.

For some reason the culminating scene, meant to out-dazzle all that went before, was felt to fall rather flat in its intended triumph. But it was placed at the end of an evening which had already stretched far into the night. Indeed, the fatigued critic of *Punch* suggested that the pantomime might, the following year, be drastically curtailed so that the audience could rely on leaving for home by 11 p.m. Yet the opinions of critics played no part in Joseph Merrick's responses, and it could for him all have gone on for ever. For Frederick Treves, on the other hand, it must have marked the end of a very long day indeed, since he had no doubt risen at his usual hour of five in the morning. He still, moreover, had the responsibility of smuggling Joseph out of the theatre again and into his closed carriage before escorting him safely home to Whitechapel.

Time did nothing to fade the glow of Joseph Merrick's bewitchment during the weeks that followed his visit to the pantomime. He would talk of it continually, and relive each ephemeral moment. As with the faculty of make-believe in childhood, so, said Treves, every aspect of the pantomime was real to him.

... the palace was the home of kings, the princess was of royal blood, the fairies were as undoubted as the children in the street, while the dishes at the banquet were of unquestionable gold. He did not like to discuss it as a play, but rather as a vision of some actual world.

The life of the pantomime story thus for Joseph went on living, even though he was no longer there to witness it. 'I wonder what the prince did after we left?' he would ask Treves among a host of similar questions. Or, 'Do you think that poor man is still in the dungeon?'

There may have been other visits to the theatre for Joseph, though no confirmation exists for those beyond an incidental remark made in a later letter to *The Times* which Carr Gomm wrote after Joseph's death. But it seems unlikely that anything he may have seen subsequently could have matched the intensity of his first experience of the living theatre.

CHAPTER 10

What Was the Matter
with Joseph Merrick?

The question of the diagnosis of Joseph Merrick's puzzling condition was last left in the hands of the dermatologist Dr Henry Radcliffe Crocker (on pages 51-2), when, in 1885, he made his tentative but positive suggestions to the meeting of the Pathological Society of London. Joseph was probably never aware of the fact that, three years further on, in 1888, he came to rest in a firm niche in medical history with the publication of Radcliffe Crocker's *magnum opus*, a two-volume work entitled *Diseases of the Skin: An Analysis of Fifteen Thousand Cases of Skin Disease*. It was destined to be a classic among medical textbooks, and the second volume contained a section on the rare group of skin diseases known as the fibromas. It was here that he inevitably mentioned the Elephant Man.

An extraordinary case of this kind was brought to the Pathological Society by Treves. I had an opportunity of examining the patient there, and at a show where he was exhibited as an 'elephant man'.

Like Tuckett, Bland-Sutton and Treves, Crocker had therefore made his pilgrimage to the freakshop in the Whitechapel Road. (Really Tom Norman had done not at all badly: he persuaded at least four doctors to pay a fee for the privilege of examining a case.) In his textbook, Crocker's technical description continued:

The bulk of the disease was on the right side; there was enormous hypertrophy of the skin of the whole right arm, measuring twelve inches round the wrist and five inches round one of the fingers, a lax mass of pendulous skin, etc., depending from the right pectoral region. The right side of the face was enormously thickened, and in addition there were huge unsymmetrical exostoses on the forehead and the occiput. There were also tumours affecting the right side of the gums and palate; on both legs, but chiefly the right, and over nearly the whole of the back and buttocks; the skin was immensely thickened, with irregular lobulated masses of confluent tumours, presenting the ordinary molluscous characters. The left arm and hand were small and well formed. The man was twenty-five years old, of stunted growth, and had a right talipes equinus, but was fairly intelligent. The disease was not perceived at birth, but began to develop when five years old, and had gradually increased since; it was, of course, ascribed to maternal fright during pregnancy.

Before saying what was the matter with Joseph Merrick, it is probably easier to say what most positively was not. To begin with, it was not the clinical condition usually labelled elephantiasis. The show name of 'The Elephant Man' which his managers chose for him has often had the unfortunate effect of leading writers into making a mis-diagnosis and assuming that elephantiasis was responsible. It has therefore been the disease cited for Joseph Merrick in a number of apparently authoritative sources, but elephantiasis is a complaint caused by a parasitic, hair-like worm which invades the body's lymphatic channels. It occurs only in tropical or sub-tropical regions, is transmitted to man through mosquito bites, and has entirely different features from those characteristic in Joseph's example.

Joseph himself, of course, was never in any doubt over what had been the cause of his great misfortune. His distorted body was for him attributable directly to the frightening experience his mother suffered while making her way through the crowded streets at the time of Leicester's Humberstonegate Fair. In *The Natural History of Nonsense*, Bergen Evans comments:

Once conception has been accomplished a further set of delusions obtain. Chief of these is the belief that certain impressions made on the mother during her pregnancy will affect the child. Of late years it has been held that pleasant impressions will have a beneficial effect and that the expectant mother should therefore keep herself cheerful, listen to good music, and frequent art galleries.

Beliefs in the imprinting of maternal impressions on unborn children are ever-present in folklore, from earliest times and in all cultures. As Mr Evans indicates, however, seeking for benign effects is only one aspect, and traditionally it was also the avoidance of undesirable or even malevolent consequences that needed to be taken into account at every step by vulnerable pregnant women. As Dr Károly Viski says in *Hungarian Peasant Customs*:

> The young woman must not hide a leaf in her bosom, because a similar mark will show on the child's breast; fruit should not fall on her, and if it does, she must not make a sudden move to catch it, as that will result in the mark of that fruit on the child. It is unwise to throw meat in the direction of the woman, especially liver, because in that case the child will get freckles.

In her study, *East Anglian Folklore*, Enid Porter records how the eating of strawberries was and is believed in this area of Britain to be the cause of a strawberry-coloured birthmark on a baby's body. In *Cambridgeshire Customs and Folklore*, also by Enid Porter, she cites the case of a Cambridge man who was born with his hands deformed, which his mother put down to a large, strange dog having leaped up shortly before his birth and placed its paws on her stomach. Mentally retarded children born in East Anglia during the Second World War were often thought to be a consequence of their mothers being startled during bombing raids. In the Cambridgeshire fens, pregnant women would traditionally try to avoid the sight of a chimney sweep in case their babies were born black-skinned.

International folklore is rich in such material, and even in the most sophisticated urban environment the folklorist would not have to search far before he found similar current examples. The belief that a fear of spiders can be transmitted to a child in this way remains remarkably common, as does the belief that spilling a cup of tea or coffee over the mother's stomach can cause birthmarks in her unborn child. That modern medical science and Bergen Evans define such notions as nonsense will matter little to those who believe them. They may even be helpful to some mothers in modifying the emotional guilt that is unfortunately so often present where a blemished or malformed baby comes into the world. In any case, it is only quite recently that medical science has rejected these beliefs. Before that, over the centuries since the time of Hippocrates, maternal impression was an integral part of a physician's advice to mothers-to-be.

The ancient Greeks advised pregnant women to gaze on statues of Castor and Pollux and other objects of great beauty so that their children might be born fair and graceful. For similar motives, pregnant ladies in nineteenth-century Paris would spend many hours in the Louvre, perambulating gently through the galleries.

In the sixteenth century, a great French doctor of the Renaissance period, Ambroise Paré, listed maternal impression among the thirteen causes for the births of abnormal children. Two hundred years later in London, however,

William Hunter, who helped to raise obstetrics to a recognized branch of medicine, approached the belief with a more questioning attitude. He carefully cross-examined the expectant mothers who came under his care for details of emotional shocks suffered since conceiving. In no example did he come across a malformation or abnormality attributable to psychic injury. He did notice, though, that whenever a small foetal abnormality occurred, the mother would have little difficulty in searching her memory to find an incident to explain the fault.

But the rational William Hunter, in remaining sceptical of the theory of maternal impression, was well ahead of his time. The belief only lost ground during the nineteenth century as medicine began to find a more securely scientific and empirical base. It came to be pointed out that perfectly normal babies are often born to mothers who have been through appalling emotional crises; that, in any case, few mothers could hope to live through a gestation period of nine months without encountering some of the shocks normal to the business of living; and yet that a majority of babies is born unmarked.

As research came to confirm, most malformations of the foetus appear before the end of the third month in pregnancy, while most events described by mothers happened during the later stages. Furthermore, no means could be discovered by which a nervous trauma might be transferred to the personality of the unborn child, for no nerve connection exists between mother and foetus, nor even an intermingling of bloodstreams.

More than at any other time in its history, the medical profession is aware today of the hazards that can damage a baby in the womb. It seems no more than common sense to advise an expectant mother to avoid certain drugs as well as serious emotional stress so far as possible, and that any maternal infection should be referred to her doctor without delay. Yet where medical science is concerned, the ancient theory of maternal impression, with its essentially magical linking of cause and effect, can safely be left to the attentions of the folklorist. We do not need to fall back on an old wives' tale to account for Joseph Merrick's complaint.

At the time when he was first examined, there were, however, considerable problems of classification, and several factors made the situation perplexing. The first and most important source of confusion was the simple fact that the disorder concerned had not as yet been completely described or labelled. A second difficulty lay in its nature, since it involved a condition capable of manifesting itself in many different ways, so that it was unlikely that any two cases, selected at random, would bear the slightest resemblance to one another in either appearance or clinical history. A third factor lay in the extreme rarity of the disorder in its more striking forms.

From the vantage point of the later decades of the twentieth century, when we have a far wider if still incomplete understanding of the disorder from which Joseph suffered, it is possible to place the problem of diagnosis in the 1880s more precisely in context. It was rather as if Treves and his contemporaries had been trying to comprehend the picture of a disease which had been broken up into a jigsaw puzzle, pieces of which were widely scattered about the world. No individual doctor was likely to find himself in possession of more than a couple of pieces of the jigsaw at any one time; he would be even less likely to know about other pieces of the puzzle, or to realize that the two or so pieces he held or knew about were related to each other, let alone were fragments of a far larger, as yet amorphous picture. That Treves, with the prompting of Radcliffe Crocker, succeeded in linking three major pieces of the puzzle and quite accurately connecting the condition with the central nervous system was an advertisement for the high standard of British medicine in 1885. It is today generally accepted that Joseph should be classified as a sufferer from neurofibromatosis, otherwise known as multiple neurofibromatosis or von Recklinghausen's disease.

Friedrich Daniel von Recklinghausen (1833–1910) was among Germany's most distinguished pathologists, the professor of pathology at the then newly founded University of Strasbourg. He was a keen observer of disease processes, and was the first to describe several different conditions with which his name is linked. In 1882, two years before Joseph was exhibited before the Pathological Society of London, von Recklinghausen gave the first description of a hitherto unrecognized disorder. It was characterized by the presence of types of tumour called neurofibromas, in connection with the nerve trunks, as well as soft, lumpy tumours of the skin and areas of cutaneous pigmentation. He noted no other abnormality and suggested no cause for its origin.

Whether Treves or Radcliffe Crocker had come across von Recklinghausen's monograph at that stage of the story's unfolding is impossible to say, but even if they had done it seems highly unlikely that they could have linked the Elephant Man with the cases being described in Strasbourg, the manifestations in Joseph's example being so bizarre and gross. Indeed, it seems most improbable that a diagnosis could have been made even if Professor von Recklinghausen himself had been able to make a first-hand examination.

The name neurofibromatosis by which the disease is known today simply means that there is a tendency in patients who suffer from it towards the formation of one or more tumours of a particular type. The kind of tumour involved is that known as a neurofibroma (one composed exclusively of a dense proliferation of nerve and fibrous tissue). Such tumours may occur singly or in great numbers within many different tissues of the body, and they can vary between the size of a pin's head and an orange. It is the extreme variability in site, size and number of tumours that accounts for the variations of symptoms in individual patients. Despite their random nature, however, it is the tendency to form neurofibromas that remains the consistent abnormality to be found in every patient in whom the disorder is diagnosed.

Most commonly, the neurofibromas form within the layers of skin, and even here their appearance may be highly variable. In the disorder's mildest forms, there will be nothing visible but a degree of skin pigmentation, taking the form of patches of skin colouring of a pale coffee shade, and these may vary from mere dots to areas the width of a man's hand. Occasionally the pigmentation may occur as diffuse shading on one or both flanks. It is unusual to find any case of the disease in which these cutaneous discolorations are not present in one form or another.

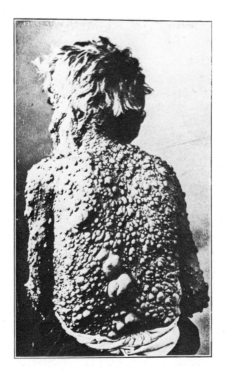

Plate 60. A case of neurofibromatosis illustrated in an 1894 medical textbook. The victim was a Hindu who considered that the thick growth of tumours had been visited on him because of a change in his religious opinions

A more severe manifestation of neurofibromatosis in the skin comes about when the fibromas form themselves into soft swellings which may or may not be pendulous and can vary between being tiny warty prominences and swellings as large as a clenched fist. These are often present in large numbers on the trunk, but also, not uncommonly, develop on the face. Treves described tumours like these in great profusion in the notes which he made on Joseph Merrick's disorder.

The most extreme skin changes of all come about when forms of diffuse tumour develop within the network of nerve fibres within the skin. These then become associated with a thickening of the skin and subcutaneous tissue, so that large folds of skin are formed; or there may be a diffuse enlargement of the subcutaneous tissues of a limb. This is a change which most usually affects the flesh overlying the temple, cheek, upper lid and back of the neck.

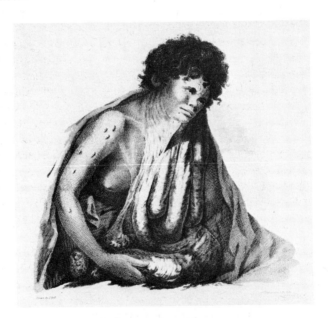

Plate 61. What may well have been a severe case of neurofibromatosis was described and illustrated in John Bell's *Principles of Surgery*, vol. 3 (1815). This 'Elephant Woman', whose name was given as 'Eleanor Fitzgerald', suffered from dramatic pendulous tumours which had to be supported if they were not to dip down almost to the ground. She, too, displayed her disfigurements in an attempt to earn her living

It was dramatic illustrations of the disease like these which Dr Radcliffe Crocker and his mentor, Dr Tilbury Fox, were citing when they spoke of dermatolysis and pachydermatocoele (see earlier, page 52). In fact, this was the technical description which continued to be applied to Joseph Merrick's case over many years, for it was not realized that such cases could be explained as extreme manifestations of the milder forms of the syndrome described by von Recklinghausen. By 1909, the link had been achieved. In that year Dr Parkes Weber, a physician to the German Hospital in London and something of a connoisseur of rare diseases, wrote in an article on von Recklinghausen's disease for the *British Journal of Dermatology*: 'The most famous example of the class was undoubtedly the famous Elephant Man whom many must have seen when he was at The London Hospital.'

In the fatty, subcutaneous tissues of the bodies of the more sorely afflicted, the neurofibromas develop as firm nodules on the trunks of the peripheral nerves so that they may be felt as tender, bead-like swellings in the limbs and on the sides of the neck. Wherever nervous tissue is found in the body, there the neurofibromas are capable of forming, and they commonly crop up on the roots of the great nerves and within the skull and the actual spinal canal.

On the face of it, it seems curious that solid structures like the bones should ever become involved. It is therefore not surprising that this connection was one of the later pieces of the jigsaw to fall into place. Only at about the turn of the century did associated bone changes come to be recognized, as when, in 1901, Jonathan Hutchinson presented the case of a woman who suffered from involvement and overgrowth of the frontal bone of the skull with the presence of bony tumours. And, in 1906, Dr Cooper reported similar findings in a young girl. Such skeletal distortions were usually found to underlie the diffuse types of skin tumour like those Joseph had exhibited. It seems certain that he was the very first patient who displayed them to be recorded.

Yet it was not until as late as 1930 that Dr Parkes Weber put forward the suggestion that the bone malformations occurred as a result of the involvement in neurofibroma formation of the periosteum (the fibrous membrane which shapes and forms the surface layers of a bone). Once again, Joseph Merrick was cited, Dr Weber remarking in his paper:

> The famous Elephant Man ... whom I once saw, and who died at The London Hospital at the age of twenty-seven years on April 11th, 1890, had many deformities of nature of pachydermatocoeles as well as many bony thickenings and outgrowths ... Irregular periosteal neurofibromatosis may well have played a part in his osseous deformities.

During the past fifty years, a number of other manifestations of neurofibromatosis have been recognized, and tumour formation or clinical abnormality has been described in practically every tissue and organ of the body. Changes have been found to take place in such varied sites as the intestines, internal glands, including the adrenals, the kidneys, and the retina of the eye. It is quite possible that varieties of the disease exist which are yet to be recognized.

The unified picture of the disease is, however, still exclusively how it appears to the pathologist or medical scientist. From the point of view of the patient or a doctor in general practice, the disorder presents yet a different aspect. To start with, it is not especially common. A doctor in general practice might expect to come across no more than two or three cases during the course of his working life.

The important point is that, in the vast majority of examples, the disorder is so minor as to cause little in the way of symptoms – perhaps a small, soft swelling that can be felt beneath the skin, or a few warty pimples hidden from sight beneath normal clothes, or a patch of lightly pigmented skin, so that the condition may be ignored or never even brought to the attention of a medical practitioner. The late Dr Richard Brasfield and Dr Tapas Das Gupta noted in their series of 110 patients seen with the disorder at the Abraham Lincoln School of Medicine, Chicago, Illinois, that twenty of their patients had sought advice only for cosmetic reasons, while in a further twenty-five instances it had been diagnosed as an incidental finding when the patient attended a doctor with some other complaint. Cases which suffer from disturbances severe enough to incommode a patient or threaten his well-being are considerable medical rarities and widely scattered.

Neurofibromatosis in fact turns up in a wide range of races and in virtually every corner of the world. As we have seen, evidence of it may be present at birth or it may make its first appearance during early childhood, though relatively few patients come under active medical care during this time. In many instances, the disease does not progress, but remains stationary for year after year. Only in the most occasional patient will it turn progressive so that each year of life sees some fresh affliction.

Some among this most unfortunate minority of patients will die from a malignant transformation occurring in one of their many tumours; in others their situation may become terminal after the growth of a neurofibroma within the skull or spinal canal; still others will succumb to an incidental

Plates 62a–c (opposite and overleaf). The distortions to the bones of Merrick's skull

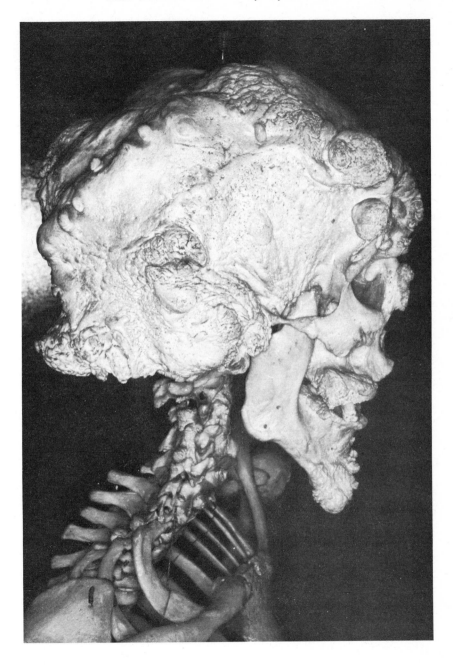

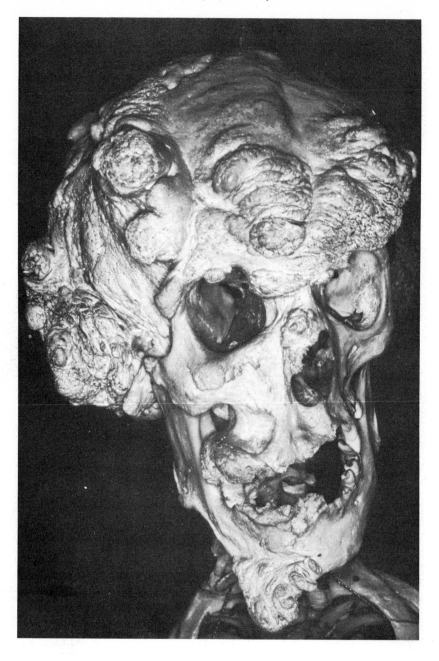

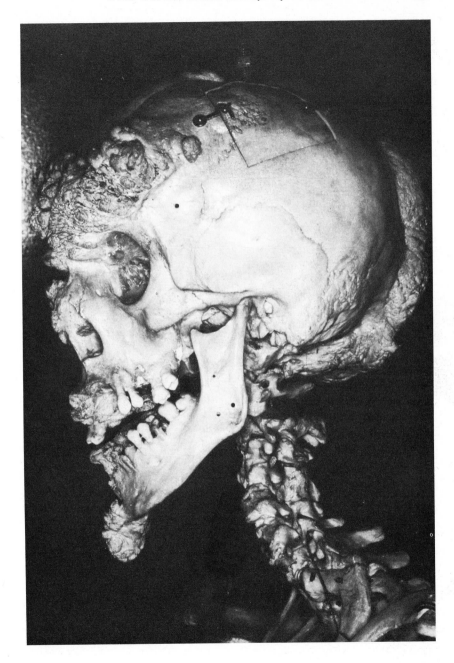

infection, tuberculosis, or simply following a period of bodily deterioration which becomes terminal. Should these ultimate dangers be avoided, other discomforts remain to harass them. In the general run of patients, as many as 12 per cent suffer from epileptic types of convulsion, and at least 10 per cent show evidence of mental retardation. In one series of cases, it was found that only 23 per cent of patients had an IQ of over 90, and in another large group of patients examined in the United States, only two individuals in the whole group had managed to complete a college education.

Quite early on in the study of neurofibromatosis, it was recognized that it could run in families, often passing over two, three or even four generations. In fact, about half of all known cases have been found to have inherited the disorder directly from an affected parent. In the other half of cases, it seems as though the disorder is sporadic, no previous case being detectable in the family tree.

Perhaps the most comprehensive study of the genetics of neurofibromatosis was that made in the University of Michigan in the early 1950s by F.W. Crowe, W.J. Schull and J.F. Neel. Their findings, published in their monograph, *Multiple Neurofibromatosis*, cleared up many problems in understanding the inheritance of the condition. At the outset, they evolved a clinical method for identifying individuals who had the disease in even its mildest forms. This was based on careful measurement and counting of areas of skin pigmentation, and they called the method the 'six-spot test'. Using it, they were then able to study the passage of the disease through many families.

Where the disease was obviously a familial complaint, they showed decisively that the disorder was inherited as a simple Mendelian dominant characteristic. In other words, in the families concerned, the disease had been invariably passed down from sufferer to sufferer without skipping a generation. Moreover, wherever such a sufferer from the disease became a parent, about half the children of the marriage showed symptoms and half were normal. The affected children were then liable to pass the disorder on yet again to the following generation in the same proportion, though the normal children could rest confident that their descendants would not do so.

One interesting point which Crowe, Schull and Neel discovered was that the disorder is not in practice transmitted as freely as might be thought, for many of the sufferers did not marry, and those who did seemed relatively infertile. Sexual and general physical underdevelopment is certainly a recognized feature of the condition in a proportion of victims.

The Michigan doctors were also able to throw some light on the origin of the sporadic cases which occur without any previous trace being present in their families. These patients were also prone to avoid marriage, and, where they did marry, also proved comparatively infertile. Where, however, the research team managed to examine thirty-five children resulting from such marriages, they found that eighteen of them, or almost half, showed evidence of the disease. Obviously, even in the sporadic cases, the disease can then become inheritable.

There is no way of knowing in precisely what manner Mary Jane Merrick, Joseph's mother, was crippled, but it seems improbable that the cause of her infirmity can have been von Recklinghausen's disease. For lack of better evidence, Joseph Carey Merrick must therefore be regarded as one of the sporadic cases of neurofibromatosis caused by a chance genetic mutation. But from the moment that he came under the care of the London Hospital, the Elephant Man has posed an endlessly fascinating puzzle for the medical world. Many eminent physicians have been tempted to hazard various and complicated diagnoses. As recently as the summer of 1982, X-ray photographs were taken of his skeleton, and these confirmed the presence of neurofibromatosis and the old childhood damage to his left hip. In studying these plates, however, Benjamin Felson, Professor of Radiology of the University of Cincinnati Hospitals, thought that he could see evidence for yet another very rare disorder that goes under the label of polyostotic fibrous displasia, and raised the possibility that this might in some way be related to neurofibromatosis.

There is little more that can or need be said about the clinical technicalities of Joseph's condition. Though the disease from which he suffered so drastically and dramatically is still not fully understood and many sufferers from its erratic range of disorders have been recognized, the fact remains that the great consensus of medical opinion considers him to be among the very worst afflicted victims of the disorder ever to have lived. In generation after generation of great medical textbooks – works of basic authority, such as Kinnier Wilson's *Neurology*, Boyd's *Textbook of Pathology*, Russell Brain's *Diseases of the Nervous System* – his name has been advanced as the supreme example of a case of multiple neurofibromatosis.

One final melancholy fact should be recorded: multiple neurofibromatosis is still incurable and hardly any more treatable than it was almost a century ago. There is, however, a concise creed that doctors through the ages have attempted to follow: to cure sometimes; to relieve often; to comfort always. Frederick Treves was not able to cure or relieve Joseph Merrick's medical state, but ultimately he did not fail his patient. If Joseph were to come among us today, our doctors and specialists could do very little more than Treves achieved in curing or relieving his sufferings.

It has become the fashion to scorn the philanthropic impulses exploited to secure Joseph's future in the London Hospital. But it is, at the same time, chastening to reflect on how society's attempts at the management of the acutely deprived and disabled in our own day would compare, both in terms of the degree of inner security and the individual standards of kindness and comfort that Treves brought to bear in the case of Joseph Merrick, though it was necessary for him to break the rules to do so.

CHAPTER 11

The Burden Falls Away

The progressive decline of Joseph Merrick was something Treves could only watch with helpless concern. From time to time he would intrude upon Joseph to make further clinical examinations and to chart the aggressive advances the disease was achieving. The bony masses and the pendulous flaps of skin continued to grow, and the stump in the upper jaw where the 'trunk' was once amputated at the Leicester Infirmary did not remain dormant but began to enlarge again, forcing Joseph's mouth into new, bizarre distortions. The intelligibility of his speech once more deteriorated. He suffered from bouts of bronchitis and the doctors knew that his heart was no longer sound. They knew, too, that he must in the end succumb to his peculiarly fungating disorder, and assumed that the end, when it came, would be sharp and sudden, perhaps in the eruption of a violent pneumonia, or following a rapid failing of the weakened heart.

There were even further confrontations with the hospital photographer. The last of the photographs, probably taken in 1888, showed the premature ageing effect for which the encroaching disease was responsible. In the space of the five years during which he had known him, Treves had seen Joseph's appearance change from that of a youth to one of an elderly man. Having reached the period of his late twenties he was entering into his old age.

Yet, despite the slow and relentless deterioration to which he was subjected, the Elephant Man seemed able to maintain an inner calm and contentment. The patient's days settled into a steady routine of reading, of receiving friends, of greeting those who passed in Bedstead Square. The daily baths and the ministrations of the nurses also punctuated the quiet hours which he spent alone with his thoughts. His mind meanwhile turned more

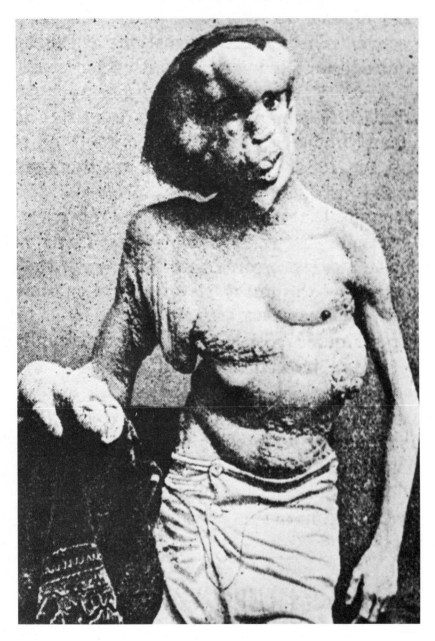

Plate 63. Joseph Merrick photographed in about 1888

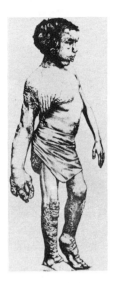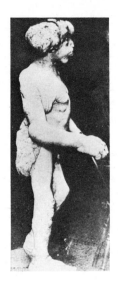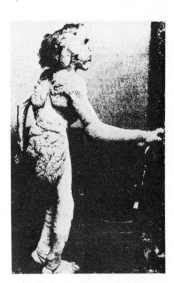

Plate 64. The rapid ageing effects of Merrick's condition are dramatically illustrated by comparing these pictures which date respectively from (a) 1884, (b) 1886 and (c) about 1888

and more in the direction of religious questions, the devotional upbringing which he received from his mother beginning to reassert its influence. In this connection he welcomed the visits of the hospital chaplain, the Rev. Tristram Valentine, who naturally encouraged his questings into simple theology.

Mr Valentine suggested that it would be perfectly possible for him to attend the hospital chapel services on Sundays, for he could sit unseen in the vestry but still hear and take part in the service. In fact Mr Valentine must have been something of a contrast to the Baptist ministers whom Joseph knew in his childhood, having a reputation for being a rather 'high' church-man. Nevertheless Joseph sought his advice and instruction, and eventually asked to be prepared for confirmation into the Anglican Church. Confirmation, of course, is a ceremony that may only be performed by a bishop, and then only after the prelate has satisfied himself that the candidate is suitable by giving an examination on the catechism. If Joseph was to be confirmed, the services of a bishop willing to meet and confirm Joseph in a private ceremony at the London Hospital needed to be obtained.

It so happened that the bishopric of London was assisted at this time in its heavy diocesan responsibilities by the suffragan bishopric of Bedford, origin-ally created by Henry VIII but fallen into disuse until its renewal in the

1870s. Dr William Walsham How, a country parson from Shropshire, was then appointed to the suffragan see, though Dr How was no routine parish priest. He took an essentially practical view of his commitments as a Christian, had a strong gift for the written and spoken word, and was a scholar in natural history and biology. Several of his hymns are still retained in the *English Hymnal,* including the processional, 'For All the Saints Who From Their Labours Rest'.

During his twenty-eight years as a parish priest in Shropshire, he had declined offers of bishoprics in various parts of the British Empire, as well as certain well-upholstered livings at home at which any more career-orientated priest might have been expected to leap. In the end he was only drawn to London by the conviction that there was work to be done among the desperately deprived lives of the people of the East End. He saw himself, in fact, as the East End's unofficial bishop, and worked tirelessly to raise funds for his poverty-stricken parishes by holding public meetings in the West End and the richer towns of southern England.

The London Hospital, of course, lay within one of those parishes. He was associated with its work and had already met Joseph Merrick, having been present there in May 1887 to offer the blessing during the ceremonies when the Prince and Princess of Wales opened the new Nurses Home and Medical College accommodation. When Mr Valentine went to the suffragan bishop with the problem of Joseph's confirmation, Dr How felt no reservations about his suitability. In due time Joseph was confirmed during a quiet private ceremony conducted within the hospital chapel.

Towards the end of his essay, Treves mentioned one other aspiration which, he said, had 'stirred the depths' of Joseph's mind: that he might visit the countryside to observe nature and experience it at first hand, after having read so much about it in books.

The country as viewed from a wagon on a dusty high road [said Treves] was all the country he knew. He had never wandered among the fields nor followed the windings of a wood. He had never climbed to the brow of a breezy down. He had never gathered flowers in a meadow.

Dame Madge Kendal mentions that Lady Dorothy Nevill, who was one of Joseph's visitors as well as a benefactor of the London Hospital, offered Joseph 'a cottage on her estate for some weeks, on condition that he did not leave it till after dark'. Whether this conditional offer on the part of a descendant of Sir Robert Walpole was ever taken up we do not know. A similar offer by Lady Louisa Knightley, however, was indeed accepted, and took place, according to Treves, during the closing months of the Elephant Man's life.

Lady Knightley's private estate was Fawsley Park, situated near Northampton, and here Joseph could have the run of a cottage without restriction. The difficulties which always came into play the moment it was necessary for Joseph to travel, however, meant that on this occasion arrangements needed to be more elaborate than usual. Treves describes how Joseph, in his accustomed style, left the London Hospital concealed within the depths of a carriage with the blinds drawn. At the main-line railway terminus a whole second-class railway carriage was reserved for his use, being run into the sidings so that he could board it unobserved away from the departure platform. Then, with blinds down, the carriage was shunted into the station to be attached to the main-line train. At Northampton, the procedure was reversed, and once again safely concealed in a cab, Joseph was brought to Fawsley Park.

Considering that so much had been achieved, with so much attention to detail, it was an irony that there should have been a breakdown of arrangements as he arrived at his destination. It was planned that he was to stay in a small cottage as guest of one of the estate workers and his wife, who would see to all his needs. Unfortunately, the wife of the house was insufficiently prepared for her visitor's appearance. As with other women who suddenly came face to face with Joseph unawares, the first glimpse proved devastating. The moment she saw Joseph being ushered into her home, the poor woman turned and fled, her apron over her head, to hide in the fields. When at last she was calmed down, it remained obvious that she was not going to be able to cope with looking after the Elephant Man. A gamekeeper's cottage lay close to the border of a small wood on the estate, and here Joseph was taken. The gamekeeper and his wife, obviously people of more robust clay, greeted Joseph with kindness and offered their hospitality.

In his account, Treves says that Merrick stayed at Fawsley for six weeks, enjoying the freedom of being able to wander unseen and unmolested about the woods since the estate was strictly preserved. He wrote several times to Treves, and his letters overflowed with descriptions of the wonders he discovered, of the trout he watched darting beneath the surface of a stream, of the wild animals he saw, of the bird-calls he heard, of his developing friendship with an apparently fierce and noisy dog. The wild flowers fascinated him, and he picked and pressed them so that he might send them to Treves to examine. Treves privately identified them as the commonest of hedgerow plants, but valued them for what they represented. They enabled him to create in words an unforgettable image of Merrick 'who had once crouched terrified in the filthy shadows of a Mile End shop ... now sitting in the sun, in a clearing among the trees, arranging a bunch of violets he had gathered'. It had all been, said Treves, 'the one supreme holiday of his life'.

Once again, however, the facts step forward to catch Treves out in poetic licence. Lady Louisa Knightley kept a diary, and this still survives in manuscript in the Northamptonshire Record Office. The earliest reference to Joseph which it contains is dated Friday, 9 September 1887, when he was evidently staying in the family of William Goodman Bird, a farmer at Haycock's Hill near the Northamptonshire village of Badby:

> Mother and I drove to Badby where two sad cases – poor old Powell dying of cancer in the face – and a young Billingham of consumption. Then on to Haycock's Hill where Joseph Merrick, the 'elephant man' about whom there has been so much in the papers, has been boarded out for some weeks with the Birds. I think it is impossible to imagine three more melancholy things – they haunt me; one can only pray – and

Plate 65. Haycock's Hill Farm, where Joseph Merrick stayed for his first country holiday under the patronage of Lady Louisa Knightley

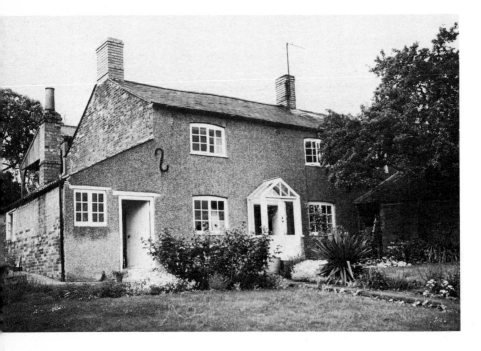

remember that Jesus lived and died for them. Merrick has such nice brown eyes! I looked straight into them – but he is *very* awful to behold. Croquet with my darling afterwards.

There is another entry for that same year, on Saturday, 29 October:

Wednesday I went again to see poor Merrick at Haycock's Hill and thence to Daventry to distribute prizes at a work show.

As a conscientious member of the upper classes, Lady Louisa Knightley struck a usual sort of balance between pursuing the social round and the performance of good works. The following year Joseph was staying at another farm in the same locality, adjoining the village of Byfield. On Wednesday, 19 September 1888, she recorded in her diary:

Mother and I went to a pleasant enough garden party at Edgcott and I visited poor Merrick by the way – and found him very comfortable and the Goldby's quite reconciled to him.

Plate 66. Redhill Farm, where he was accommodated on the next two occasions

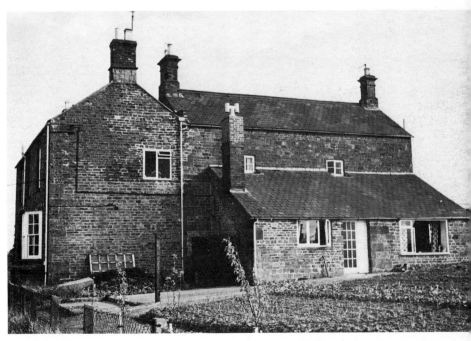

The mention of the Goldbys is interesting as it seems to be a reference to the unfortunate incident which Treves describes. That Mrs Goldby was happily able to accept Joseph in the end is borne out by one brief entry for Thursday, 5 September 1889: 'Went on the way to see poor Merrick who is at the Redhill Farm again.'

Thus it was not one but three supreme holidays which Joseph Merrick enjoyed in the Northamptonshire countryside. Mr Goldby seems in fact to have been a gamekeeper, so Treves apparently reversed the households concerned. But Redhill Farm lay just about a quarter of a mile back along the track from Redhill Wood which was skirted by the main Daventry to Banbury road, and Joseph could therefore easily have walked at leisure between the house and the woodland unobserved as Treves describes it. While at Redhill he was moreover befriended by a local farm lad called Walter Steel, who told to his family in later recollection of how he would call on him each day to chat and pick up any letters he had written to take them

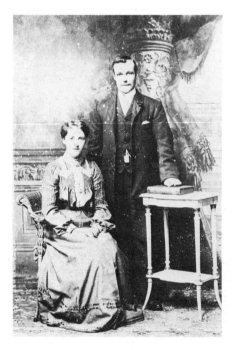

Plate 67. Walter Steel with his wife. As a farm lad, Walter had befriended the Elephant Man at Redhill

to the post. He, too, was impressed by the interesting quality of Joseph's conversation and by someone whom he felt to be a well-educated man. Mr Merrick, he remembered, composed a great many letters, and would sit out of sight in the woods to write them. He also remembered that Joseph liked to read a great deal of poetry, and spoke of the delight which he took in the natural world.

If Joseph's body was degenerating as the decade of the 1880s drew to its close, his spirit seemed somehow immune to decay; his peace of mind and quiet contentment were obvious to all who had contact with him. His life was growing more restricted, and he found it necessary to conserve his strength, making it his habit to remain in bed till midday. The afternoons he would spend reading or writing letters. The evenings were the precious moment when he chose to escape from the confinement of his rooms to walk alone, unseen in the hospital gardens.

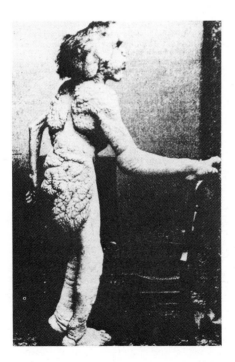

Plate 68. This photograph, one of the last taken, probably dates from 1888. Although his body had deteriorated so drastically, Joseph still had about two years to live

His spirits remained good, and on Easter Sunday, 6 April 1890, he twice attended the chapel services, taking communion in the morning. On the following Thursday evening, he walked as usual in the garden, then retired to bed. On Friday morning, 11 April, he followed his usual custom, staying in bed until noon. When his nurse, Nurse Ireland of Blizzard Ward, came to attend his needs, she spoke to him but noticed nothing in his condition to cause anxiety. She left him sitting up in bed. At 1.30 p.m. a wardmaid arrived with his lunch and left it for him to eat in his own time. And then, shortly after three o'clock, Mr Hodges, Treves's current house surgeon, came down to Bedstead Square to pay his routine call. He found the Elephant Man lying across his bed, and saw at once that he was dead. The untouched lunch remained where the wardmaid had left it.

The house surgeon felt so shaken that he thought it best to refrain from touching the body until he could obtain the help of a more senior colleague, Mr Ashe. The doctors had expected Joseph's end to be swift, but not so startlingly sudden. Only when Mr Ashe arrived was the body disturbed as the two surgeons examined Joseph together, turning him this way and that as they sought the explanation for his abrupt departure out of life.

An inquest on Joseph Merrick was held at the London Hospital on Tuesday, 15 April 1890. Mr Wynne Baxter, the coroner for Central Middlesex, heard the evidence, and next morning *The Times* carried a full report headed 'Death of The Elephant Man'.

Charles Barnabus Merrick, hairdresser, tobacconist and umbrella repairer of Churchgate, Leicester, had journeyed south to perform the last unhappy service which he could for his nephew: formally to identify his mortal remains. His uncle remained the one person in his family to have stood by Joseph so far as it was in his power. Of Joseph's natural father, only the bare fact was recorded that he was known to be still alive.

As the inquest moved on to its essential business, Mr Ashe confirmed that death had been natural.

> Witness believed that the exact cause of death was asphyxia, the back of his head being greatly deformed, and while the patient was taking a natural sleep the weight of the head overcame him, and so suffocated him.

Nurse Ireland and Mr Hodges respectively described Joseph's last hours and the finding of his body, and then the coroner summed up, saying:

> '... there could be no doubt that death was quite in accordance with the theory put forward by the doctor. The jury accepted this view and

returned a verdict that death was due to suffocation from the weight of the head pressing upon the windpipe.

In parallel, on the same day, the house committee of the London Hospital used its Tuesday meeting to discuss the problems raised by Joseph's demise. Treves offered his comments to the committee, from which medical men were rigorously excluded, and the minutes were as brisk as ever.

It was decided that the skeleton should be set up in the College Museum, a funeral service having been held in the chapel before the body was handed over to Mr Treves, the licensed anatomist of the college.

Mr Carr Gomm read a letter he proposed sending to *The Times* re Merrick and Mr Carr Gomm was thanked for his kindness in writing it.

The point was that so much interest had been aroused by the Elephant Man's plight, and so many influential benefactors had come forward to help, that the news of Joseph's death was unavoidably a matter of public concern. Carr Gomm's letter was an attempt not only to offer the world a full picture of Joseph's life and death in the care of the London Hospital, but also to make account of his stewardship of the charity he had sought on Joseph's behalf. It was printed in *The Times* of Wednesday, 16 April 1890, immediately beneath the report of the inquest. Once again it summarized at length the desperation of Joseph's life before chance brought about his admission to the London Hospital, and the generosity of the public response which enabled him to remain.

There he received kindly visits from many, among them the highest in the land, and his life was not without various interests and diversions; he was a great reader and was well supplied with books; through the kindness of a lady, one of the brightest ornaments of the theatrical profession, he was taught basket making, and on more than one occasion he was taken to the play, which he witnessed from the seclusion of a private box.

The next paragraph made much of Joseph's virtues, of his confirmation by the bishop, of his attendance at chapel services, and how, during the last conversation he had with the chaplain, he 'expressed his feelings of deep gratitude for all that had been done for him here, and his acknowledgement of the mercy of God in bringing him to this place'. Then there was the six weeks' outing which he had enjoyed at a country cottage 'each year'. Yet, declared Carr Gomm, despite 'all this indulgence' he remained 'quiet and unassuming, very grateful for all that was done for him, and conformed himself readily to the restrictions that were necessary'. Even into the very grave, Joseph Merrick's status as an infinitely deserving case needed to be emphasized over and over.

I have given these details, thinking that those who sent money to me for his support would like to know how their charity was applied. Last Friday afternoon, though apparently in his usual health he quietly passed away in his sleep.

I have left in my hands a small balance of the money which has been sent me from time to time for his support, and this I now propose, after paying certain gratuities, to hand over to the general funds of the hospital. This course, I believe, will be consonant with the wishes of the contributors.

It was the courtesy of *The Times* in inserting my letter in 1886, that procured for this afflicted man a comfortable protection during the last years of a previously wretched existence, and I desire to take this opportunity of thankfully acknowledging it.

Among those who took a personal interest in the news of Joseph's passing was Lady Louisa Knightley at Fawsley Park. She made a note of the event in her journal:

I see in today's paper that poor Merrick, the 'Elephant Man', is dead, passed quietly away in his sleep. It is a merciful way of going out of what to him has been a very sad world, though he has received a great deal of kindness in it. Thank God – he was not unprepared. Now! he is safe and at rest.

When Carr Gomm's first appeal appeared, the *British Medical Journal* had followed it up with a report on the Elephant Man. Now, on 19 April, it did the same, its informant once more being Treves himself. The report reminded readers of the earlier reference and stated that Joseph's death had occurred at 'the age of 27, according to his relatives'. This at once created a problem since the article four years before said his age was twenty-seven then. 'His age must therefore have been overstated four years ago ...' The inquest report in *The Times* created further confusion by saying he was twenty-nine, but Treves was correct in accepting the relatives' statement for the *British Medical Journal*. Joseph's age at death was in fact twenty-seven years and eight months.

He derived the name by which he was known [said the *British Medical Journal* report] from the proboscis-like projection of his nose and lips, together with the peculiar shape of his deformed forehead. His real name was John [*sic*] Merrick. He was victimized by showmen for a time; when shown in the Whitechapel Road, the police stopped the exhibition. He was afterwards exhibited in Belgium, where he was plundered of his savings. On one occasion a steamboat captain refused to take him as a passenger.

The report went on with an account of Joseph's appearance and deformities, and proceeded to 'say a few words on poor Merrick's last days and death':

> The bony masses and pendulous flaps of skin grew steadily. The outgrowths from the upper jaw and its integuments – the so-called trunk – increased so as to render his speech more and more difficult to understand. The most serious feature, however, in the patient's illness was the increasing size of the head, which ultimately caused his death. The head grew so heavy that at length he had great difficulty in holding it up. He slept in a sitting or crouching position, with his hands clasped over his legs, and his head on his knees. If he lay down flat the heavy head tended to fall back and produce a sense of suffocation.
>
> Nevertheless, the general health of the 'elephant man' was relatively good shortly before his death ... At 1.30 p.m. on Friday he was in bed (he seldom got up until the afternoon) and appeared to be perfectly well when the wardmaid brought him his dinner. Between 3 and 4 o'clock he was dead in his bed.
>
> Mr Treves, to whom we are indebted for the above details, is of the opinion that from the position in which the patient lay after death it would appear that the ponderous skull had fallen backwards and dislocated his neck.

A résumé of the inquest followed, and then, in the penultimate paragraph, there came a most interesting misstatement:

> We understand that the Committee of the London Hospital refused not only to permit a necropsy on the body of the 'elephant man', but also declined to allow his body to be preserved.

The facts of the matter were that, in the Anatomy Department of the Medical College of the London Hospital, casts had already been made of Joseph's body and the process of dissection was well under way. Unless this was a genuine misunderstanding, it is impossible to avoid the impression that Treves felt it would be unpolitic for the information to be made public. Perhaps he feared that it might create distress for those who had responded

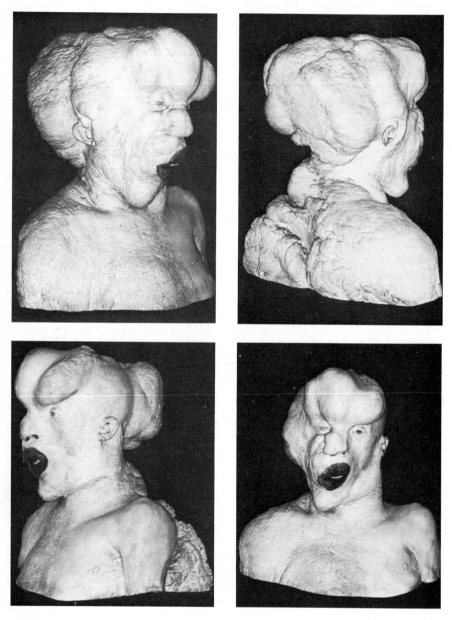

Plates 69a–d. The post-mortem cast of Merrick's head and shoulders seen from four angles

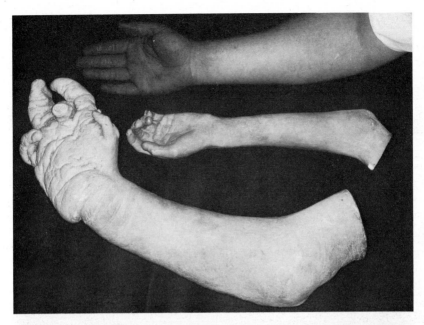

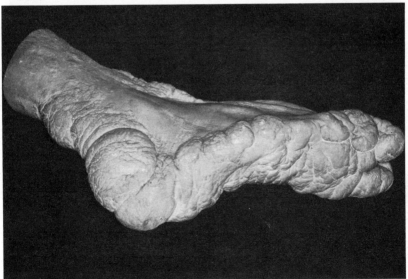

Plates 70a–b. The casts of Merrick's arms compared with a normal arm, and a cast of his foot

so compassionately in contributing to Joseph's happiness and welfare as well as, in many cases, cultivating his company.

When reading the various accounts of Joseph's end, it becomes clear that the doctors found some difficulty in explaining the eventual physical disaster which was the cause of death. There can be little doubt that Treves was the person most intimately acquainted with Joseph, and equally little doubt that he was one of the most gifted medical figures of his generation. It is probably therefore Treves's own account of Joseph's death in 'The Elephant Man' which should take precedence as the definitive version:

> ... he was found dead in his bed ... in April, 1890. He was lying on his back as if asleep, and had evidently died suddenly and without a struggle, since not even the coverlet of the bed was disturbed. The method of his death was peculiar. So large and so heavy was his head that he could not sleep lying down. When he assumed the recumbent position the massive skull was inclined to drop backwards, with the result that he experienced no little distress. The attitude he was compelled to assume when he slept was very strange. He sat up in bed with his back supported by pillows, his knees were drawn up, and his arms clasped round his legs, while his head rested on the points of his bent knees.
>
> He often said to me that he wished he could lie down to sleep 'like other people'. I think on this last night [*sic*, since as we know, he died during the early afternoon] he must, with some determination, have made the experiment. The pillow was soft, and the head, when placed on it, must have fallen backwards and caused a dislocation of the neck. Thus it came about that his death was due to the desire that had dominated his life – the pathetic but hopeless desire to be 'like other people'.

The house surgeons, coroner and death certificate all spoke of asphyxia and suffocation; Treves, in his essay and the article in the *British Medical Journal*, spoke of dislocation of the neck. But Treves, it must be said, had had the advantage of actually dissecting the body after death. He supervised the taking of the plaster casts of the head and limbs, the preservation of the skin samples (subsequently lost when their storage jar dried out during the Second World War), and finally the mounting of the bones one by one into

Plates 71a–c (opposite and overleaf). Three views of Merrick's skeleton compared with the cast of his head. In (b) it is possible to see his badly atrophied arthritic left hip joint

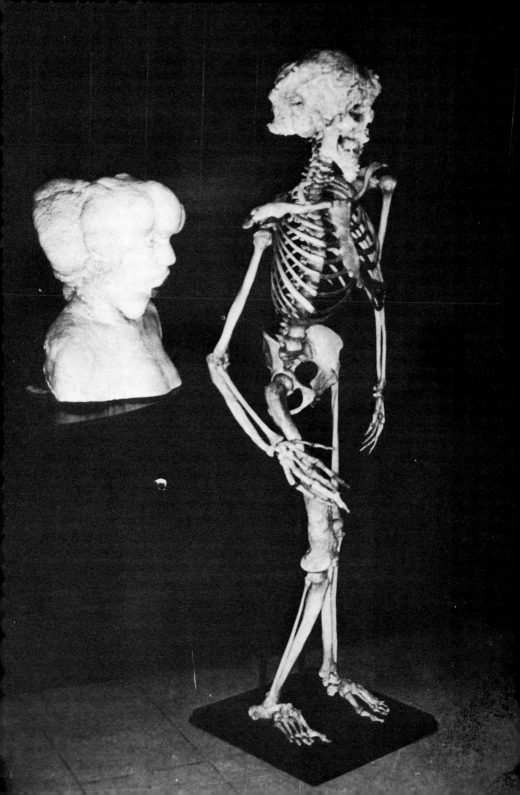

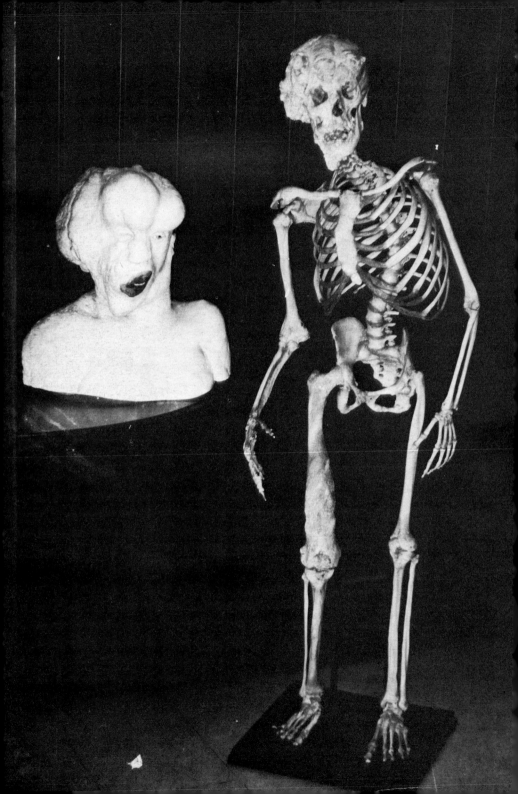

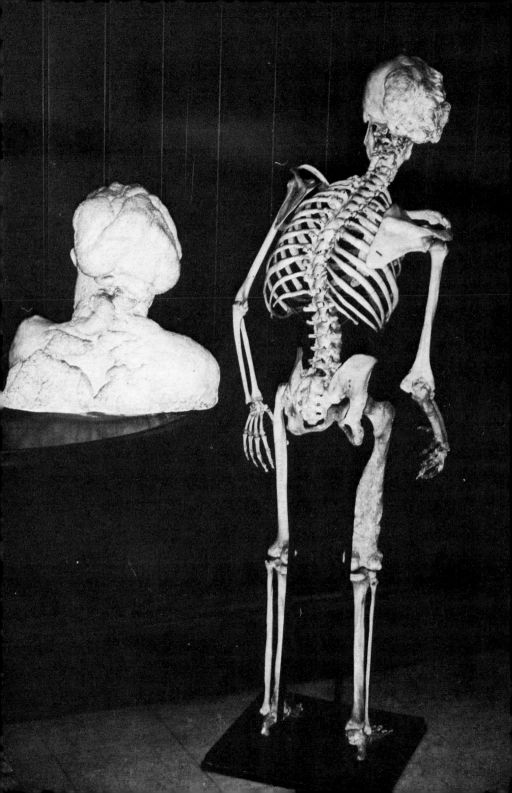

an entire skeleton. It must have been a gruesome and disturbing task, made doubly distasteful since this was for Treves the body of someone with whom he had been in a unique mixture of personal and professional relationship.

Treves, however, was too fine a doctor to mistake the flesh for the man. Writing of their first encounter, he described Joseph as 'the most disgusting specimen of humanity' that he ever saw. Towards the end of his account of the Elephant Man's life, he sought to find the words to express what he had learnt of Joseph's internal nobility.

As a specimen of humanity, Merrick was ignoble and repulsive; but the spirit of Merrick, if it could be seen in the form of the living, would assume the figure of an upstanding and heroic man, smooth browed and clean of limb, and with eyes that flashed undaunted courage.

CHAPTER 12

The Figure in Time's Fabric

As is usually the case with those who, in any sphere of life, have no fear of breaking eggs when it comes to making omelettes, Frederick Treves possessed enemies as well as friends. Those who admired him did so unstintingly, but he also had his detractors among his medical colleagues. Some considered that he built his career on a certain rather unprofessional flair for publicity, and he certainly had a notably happy knack for being in the right place at the right time. Even one of his more ardent admirers, Dr D.G. Halsted, stated in *Doctor in the Nineties* that Treves first became famous because of the care he lavished on the Elephant Man. It is only one step from a statement like this to the innuendo that he used his association with Merrick for self-advancement. Side by side with it went another: that the hospital administrators had exploited Merrick as a publicity device in their fund-raising campaigns. Meanwhile, in the streets outside, the people of the East End, mistrustful as always of the motives of authority, held for many years to the belief that the Elephant Man sold his body to the hospital in return for the care it offered him.

The public appeals made by the hospital on Joseph's behalf, and Carr Gomm's conscientious stewardship of the donated funds, make any business transaction involving the disposal of Joseph's body seem unnecessary as well as most unlikely. As for the Elephant Man's publicity value to the hospital, this no doubt existed, but was surely incidental. There is no evidence for any calculated or cynical exploitation in the dealings which the hospital and Frederick Treves had with Joseph Merrick. To the question, on the other hand, of whether Joseph's precipitate and unexpected return to the scene in 1886 contributed to the growth of Treves's fame and fortune, the reply must be: very probably, yes, it did.

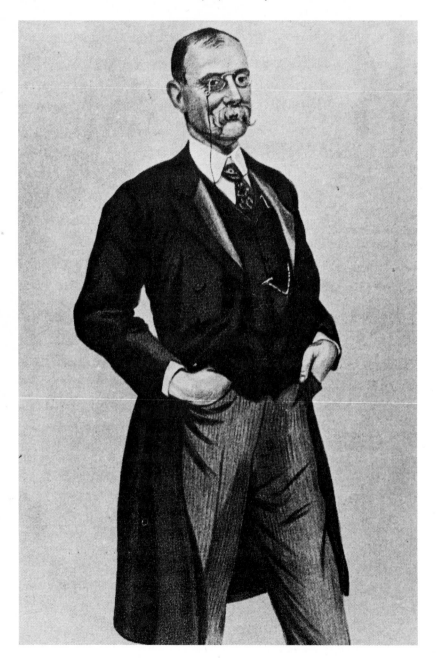

The line of development which Treves's career as a distinguished medical personality was taking was well established by the time he first met the Elephant Man. The association is unlikely to have made much difference to his ultimate professional status within the field of medicine. Yet, in the context of Treves's need to build up his private Wimpole Street surgeon's practice (his surgical duties in the public wards of the London Hospital being unpaid), the timing of Joseph's reappearance could hardly have been more opportune. It is hard to believe that the flurry of public interest which occurred in December 1886 did anything but draw his name to the attention of the rich and influential and enhance the prosperity of his practice. It may even have been an important stepping stone in bringing him to the notice of the Prince and Princess of Wales.

In other words, it must have contributed a significant momentum to Treves's financial success, but only the sternest of puritan moralists could blame him for not hesitating to accept his good fortune. The one valid question to ask is whether his success in any way compromised his integrity as a surgeon, and that it did not do so has to be the decisive answer.

There is nothing to support any accusation that he deliberately set out to utilize his knowledge of Joseph Merrick's case for financial gain. At the outset he can hardly have foreseen the course which events were to follow, and his preliminary investigations amounted to no more than a diagnostic foray to try to elucidate the cause of a mystery. Thereafter his only writings on or presentation of the case were exclusively to professional colleagues or in medical journals. Not until the last year of his life, long after his retirement from active practice, did he publish his recollections of Merrick for a more general audience in *The Elephant Man and Other Reminiscences*.

Even while Joseph was still alive, Treves was continuing to add cornerstones to his career in the shape of his medical writings. His third book, *Intestinal Obstruction: Its Varieties, with their Pathology, Diagnosis and Treatment*, based on the essay which won him the Jacksonian Prize of the Royal College of Surgeons in 1883, came from the press in 1884 and was swiftly regarded as a medical source book. The next year he produced *The Anatomy of the Intestinal Canal and Peritoneum*, based on his Hunterian Lectures, and the book represented the high point of his achievement as a surgeon writer, becoming a classic of medical literature. In 1886, he edited a three-volume textbook of surgery with contributions from thirty-five leading surgeons of the day, *A Manual of Surgery by Various Authors*.

Plate 72 (opposite). Sir Frederick Treves, the eminent man of medicine, is drawn by 'Spy' for *Vanity Fair* in 1900

After that he seems for a time to have abandoned the pen to concentrate more on the scalpel. A young engineer was admitted to the London Hospital in December 1886, suffering from typhlitis, as appendicitis was then known. The generally prescribed treatment at the time was complete bed rest, with doses of opium to relieve the pain and enemas to relieve the bowels. The engineer recovered after six weeks, but it was known that the condition would inevitably recur, and that next time it could be fatal. Treves was therefore consulted to see if he could suggest an alternative treatment, and he recommended surgery. It was a controversial and bold decision in so far as medical orthodoxy considered that acute typhlitis should simply be allowed to run its course.

When he opened up his patient, Treves found the trouble lay in a kinking of the appendix which was trapping mucus and leading to inflammation. As Treves prepared to remove the appendix and freed the peritoneal folds (the layers of membrane which line the abdominal cavity), the appendix sprang back into its normal position. Treves therefore simply sewed his patient up again, and the man duly recovered, though he was kept under anxious observation for nearly two months. There was no recurrence of typhlitis in the engineer, and, so far as is known, this was the first operation undertaken in Britain to treat chronic, relapsing appendicitis. It made Treves a leading authority in this particular branch of surgery.

Meanwhile Treves's reputation as a surgeon spread far and wide in fashionable circles. Sir Henry Irving consulted him when he inhaled the nozzle of a throat spray into his lung. He performed a desperate tracheotomy by the light of an oil lamp on the Victorian painter and president of the Royal Academy, Sir John Millais, who was a victim of throat cancer. Another rich patient, a Mr Fielden, donated £22,000 to the London Hospital in gratitude for what Treves had been able to do for him. The hospital built a complete isolation block on the strength of it, and Mr Fielden then made further donations of £62,000, and left the hospital £100,000 in his will.

In the 1890s, Treves resumed his medical authorship, producing in 1891 a large, two-volume textbook, *A Manual of Operative Surgery*, concerned solely with the practical aspects of treatment by operation. An abridged version followed a year later, and in 1895 his last full-length medical textbook, *A System of Surgery*, also in two volumes, was published. He was writing these during an intensely busy period during which he continued to fulfil his duties as consulting surgeon to the London Hospital. In fact he did not resign from his post there until 1898, the year after Queen Victoria's Diamond Jubilee celebrations.

A sequence of personal honours was now the inevitable corollary of the advances in his career. Following the outbreak of the Boer War in 1899, he saw service in South Africa as a surgeon to one of the field hospitals. He witnessed the relief of Ladysmith, but then a severe bout of dysentery laid him low. While he was still recovering, the Court Circular announced that Queen Victoria had been pleased to appoint Mr Treves as one of her surgeons-in-ordinary. Within the year the queen was dead and the Prince of Wales had succeeded to the throne as Edward VII. On 4 May 1901 the following announcement appeared in the Court Circular:

> Mr Frederick Treves was introduced to the King's presence when His Majesty conferred upon him the honour of Knighthood and invested him with the insignia of a Knight Commander of the Royal Victorian Order. Sir Frederick Treves who was Surgeon in Ordinary to her late Majesty Queen Victoria and is Surgeon in Ordinary to the Duke of Cornwall and York was recently appointed one of the honorary Sergeant Surgeons to the King.

Since the Royal Victorian Order is awarded personally by the monarch, and for services only to the sovereign and his or her family, it might have seemed that Treves was at the apogee of his ambitions. Yet, only a year before, a personal and ironic tragedy had struck at the family of the surgeon who was probably his country's leading expert in acute appendicitis. His younger daughter, Hetty, was struck down by the condition at the age of eighteen, and became mortally ill. He called in two eminent colleagues, but they could only gently tell him that if he could do nothing for her there was no one in the country who could do better. Her death cast a shadow for him over all the years which followed, though his most dramatic encounter with appendicitis was still to come. When Edward VII became ill almost on the eve of his coronation in June 1902, it was appendicitis which was diagnosed. As soon as it was decided that an operation on the king's appendix was imperative if his life was to be saved, and that the coronation would have to be postponed, it was Treves who stood by to make the historic cut and who drained the offending abscess, deciding it was not essential actually to remove the appendix itself. Twenty-one years later, in its obituary notice of the surgeon, *The Times* wrote:

> Though Treves had eminent colleagues who supported him, he was in principal charge and the real responsibility for the operation and postponing the Coronation rested wholly on his shoulders. Only a man of inflexible resolution, perfectly convinced of the correctness of his diagnosis and proposed treatment, could have carried it through.

In Edward VII's Coronation Honours List, Treves was one of those who received a baronetcy.

It surprised many that this was the point when, apparently at the height of his powers, Treves chose virtually to bring his medical career to an end. But, he had once said, no surgeon should operate after the age of fifty. Not that his was destined to be an idle retirement: he retained his royal appointments and became involved, among other things, as a founder member of the British Red Cross Society and in setting up the Radium Institute in London, to pioneer the uses of radium in British medicine. The wealth he had accumulated, however, meant that he had no further need to work for a living, while King Edward had granted him the use of Thatched House Lodge in Richmond Park as a home. There had always been about him something of a writer manqué, but it is hardly possible to build up a literary reputation by composing medical textbooks, however elegant their phrasing.

A book for the general market, *The Tale of a Field Hospital*, had in fact come out of a series of field dispatches which he sent home to the *British Medical Journal* from the war in South Africa, and it had met with an encouraging reception. Others were now to follow. In 1905 he published *The Other Side of the Lantern*, an often vivid collection of travel impressions accumulated from a round-the-world trip. It was reprinted five times in the year of publication. The next year he brought out his volume on Dorset for the *Highways and Byways* counties series. For over seventy years, it has remained a classic of regional topography, and to write it he visited every town, village, hamlet and manor house in the county by bicycle, pedalling a total distance of 2,200 miles.

The bonds that Treves felt for his native Dorset remained strong throughout his life. He had continued to visit the county at every opportunity, and it reciprocated his interest by electing him first president of the Dorset Society. In 1905 he took a house in Dorchester, close to Max Gate, the home of Thomas Hardy, and while there he developed a former acquaintanceship with the poet and novelist into a close friendship. The desk which Hardy used for his writing throughout his life was in fact originally bought from Treves's father's shop in the county town.

Other travel books came from Treves's pen. A trip to the Caribbean produced *The Cradle of the Deep* (1908), and one to Africa resulted in *Uganda for a Holiday* (1909). A visit to the Holy Land produced *The Land That is Desolate* (1911), and then he undertook a close study of Robert Browning's long narrative poem in an Italian setting, 'The Ring and the Book'. This he described as: 'One of the finest, most imaginative and most human poems of the nineteenth century ... Some of the passages ... are amongst the most beautiful to be found in any country or any age.' He made an expedition to Italy to work out the topography of the poem, accumulating a profusion of maps, plans and photographs. The photographs he took himself (as he did for several of his other books), and was careful to take them not only in the places described by Browning, but at the right time of day and in the right season of the year. It was all eventually published as *The Country of 'The Ring and the Book'* (1913).

The outbreak of the First World War called a temporary halt to Sir Frederick's literary efforts and he returned to official duties. Only after the war was he able to move his household to Switzerland, to live on the shores of Lake Geneva and take up his pen once more. Two more books were produced, *The Riviera on the Corniche Road* (1921) and *The Lake of Geneva* (1922). But by now his health was showing signs of giving way, and only one more book was to come. This, of course, was the title by which he was to be longest remembered, *The Elephant Man and Other Reminiscences* (1923). He was suffering by now from a weakened heart, but had recovered remarkably from a bout of severe pneumonia in 1922. In early December 1923, however, a sudden chill developed into peritonitis, and by the seventh of the month he was dead. His body was cremated at Lausanne.

The Society of Dorset Men arranged for Treves's ashes to be interred with appropriate ceremony in Dorchester cemetery, but a brief farce was yet to intervene when the customs refused to let the small container through unless they could be shown the death certificate. Treves's publisher, Newman Flower, recorded in his book *Just As It Happened* how he invoked the name of the king and obtained a special order from the Home Office to get the ashes past this bureaucratic hitch.

The ceremony was in due course held with a most distinguished gathering, but took place on a day of foul weather amid sheets of driving rain. After moving off from the house where Treves had been born, 8 Cornhill, the funeral procession moved on to St Peter's Church for a service, and then arrived at Dorchester cemetery with its host of mourners. Lord Dawson of Penn represented the royal family; Newman Flower came for Lady Treves. Thomas Hardy himself had chosen the hymns for the funeral service, and determinedly went on to stand in the exposed cemetery, shaking with cold and with the rain pouring down his face, brushing aside the pleas of those who feared it would be the death of the old man. 'I have known Treves since he was young,' he told Newman Flower, 'and I am going through with it.'

Once he was alone in his study later that night, the great writer who had transformed his native Wessex into an immortal and peopled literary landscape by his novels and poems, confided to his journal the sparest of impressions:

> January 2. Attended Frederick Treves' funeral at St Peter's. Very wet day. Sad procession to the cemetery. Casket in a little white grave.

The experience of having known Treves, however, coalesced into 'In the Evening', a poem which was published in *The Times* two days later. Eventually, in its finally revised and polished version, it was included in *Human Shows, Far Phantasies* (1925), the penultimate volume of Hardy's verse and the last to be published during his lifetime.

In the Evening
IN MEMORIAM FREDERICI TREVES, 1853–1923
(Dorchester Cemetery, Jan. 2, 1924)

In the morning, when the world knew he was dead,
    He lay amid the dust and hoar
Of ages; and to a spirit attending said:
        'This chalky bed? –
I surely seem to have been here before?'

'O yes. You have been here. You knew the place,
    Substanced as you, long ere your call;
And if you cared to do so, you might trace
        In this grey space
Your being, and the being of men all.'

Thereto said he: 'Then why was I called away?
    I knew no trouble or discontent:
Why did I not prolong my ancient stay
        Herein for aye?'
The spirit shook its head, 'None knows: you went.

'And though, perhaps, Time did not sign to you
    The need to go, dream-vision sees
How Aesculapius' phantom hither flew,
        With Galen's, too,
And his of Cos – plague-proof Hippocrates,

'And beckoned you forth, whose skill had read as theirs,
    Maybe, had Science changed to spell
In their day, modern modes to stem despairs
        That mankind bears! . . .
Enough. You have returned. And all is well.'

The warmest tribute of all, however, came from Queen Alexandra, the Queen Mother. She sent a cross composed of flowers gathered in her own garden at Sandringham, and with it a card which bore the inscription:

> For my beloved Sir Frederick Treves, whom we all loved so dearly and now miss so sadly, from his affectionate Alexandra, Sandringham, Norfolk.

More than thirty years had passed since Joseph Merrick himself found release from the burden of his earthly existence. It seems odd, perhaps even significant, that Frederick Treves should have turned back to the topic of the Elephant Man's life when he was so close to the end of his own. The first into print with a personal reminiscence of the Elephant Man was in fact Sir Wilfred Grenfell, Treves's former house surgeon, who included one paragraph on Merrick in his autobiography, *A Labrador Doctor*. Since this came out in 1920 and Treves must almost certainly have read it, perhaps it had the effect of spurring him into thinking he should write down his own version.

After Treves's essay 'The Elephant Man' was published, others who had had a personal acquaintanceship with or knowledge of Joseph Merrick included their reminiscences in various books, among them John Bland-Sutton in *The Story of a Surgeon* (1930) and Madge Kendal in *Dame Madge Kendal by Herself* (1933). All of these to some degree leaned on Treves's essay to help with prompting their own recollections. The last to publish a first-hand memory was Dr D.G. Halsted, whose *Doctor in the Nineties* (1959) arrived in the bookshops when he was himself ninety-one.

In *Just As It Happened*, Sir Newman Flower actually records an anecdote on how the surgeon author's last work came to be written. As his publisher at Cassell, Newman Flower had pressed Treves to set down some of his medical reminiscences, and when he was shown some of the work in progress felt excitedly that here was potentially the finest of all his author's books. The manuscript included a magnificently written and dramatic account of the operation on Edward VII. Unfortunately, and quite by chance, Treves happened to mention the projected work to Cassell's medical director.

'My dear Treves,' he said at once, 'you can't do this. You can't write any reminiscences. It can't be done . . .'

To Newman Flower's frustration and chagrin, he now found it impossible to shift from Treves's mind the idea that he might be inadvertently breaking proprieties concerning well-known people. The surgeon was adamant that he could not continue. Eventually he said to Flower, to placate his disappointment:

'Tell you what I'll do. I'll write you another book ... about the queer unknown patients I've had – patients from the great army of suffering men and women I've been mixed up with.'

As it turned out, *The Elephant Man and Other Reminiscences* was a set of twelve anecdotal pieces, but pride of place among those of the 'great army' who were thus lifted out of anonymity went, of course, to the Elephant Man. It has already been said that Treves, as writer and narrator, continues to deserve our respect, that he was capable of working up a sombre, even morbid and subjective power in his imagery. One interesting example of this type of his writing occurs in the travel book, *The Other Side of the Lantern*, where he includes a most unscientific description of a mangrove swamp on Singapore:

> Dead creepers hang into the gloom of this forest morgue; dead boughs block every gap and path as with the debris of some grim disaster; about the ground are dead trunks, with shrunken and contorted limbs, and bare roots in worm-like bundles, that seem to be writhing out of the ooze.
>
> In the undergrowth of this swamp of despair are horrible fungi, bloated and sodden. Some are scarlet, some are spotted like snakes, some have the pallor of a corpse. All seem swollen with venom. There are ghastly weeds, too, lank, colourless, and sapless – the seedlings of a devil's garden ...
>
> By silent and devious passages the soiled sea creeps into the swamp. It crawls in like a thief seeking to hide. When the tide is full the floor of the outcast wood is buried in fetid water; when the tide slinks out it leaves behind a reeking and evil mud, which is smeared over every bank and root like a poisonous ointment.
>
> To make complete the picture of this Slough of Despond one might fancy a hunted man in its most putrid hollow brushing the vermin from his wet rags and listening with terror to the tramp of eager feet about the margin of the mere.

It is in fact the touch of melodrama in the imagery of 'The Elephant Man' which makes it so unforgettable, and it has to be re-emphasized that the Elephant Man's story would most probably remain entirely unknown outside the specialist literature unless Treves had set it down. Yet even up to the point where he submitted the manuscript to his publisher he continued to be haunted by second thoughts over the wisdom of putting this particular story before his readership. He wrote to Newman Flower:

The story of the Elephant Man is, I suppose, unique and in the hands of a more competent writer would make very 'hot stuff' ... I beg you to be absolutely candid about it. My books have done alright so far and I don't want to end up with a failure. I read the MS through again before I sent it off and I am full of horrible doubts about it. If you say – and I am sure you will be Dorset straight about it – that it won't do I shall be almost relieved. It is no use to brag that every incident in the book is true; for I am doubtful if these are the kind of truths the public want.

Of all Treves's writings, 'The Elephant Man' is undoubtedly the one that will continue to be read long after the others are forgotten. If Treves owed Joseph Merrick a debt of sorts, he had gone a long way towards repaying it. In the air there is left hanging only one of the teasing, unanswerable questions of which history has many examples: had Frederick Treves not persisted in waiting while Mr Norman was searched out in the pub to come and open up his freakshow on that autumn day of 1884, but had given up and returned to his duties in the hospital, would he ever have found himself standing at the bedside of Edward VII, about to perform one of the most famous operations in the history of surgery?

Before leaving the subject of Treves's manuscript, it is intriguing to note that when it surfaced for auction in Sotheby's London sale rooms in July 1980, it turned out to throw one small but significant beam of light on the long-standing mystery of how it came about that Treves delivered Joseph to posterity with the wrong Christian name. In fact, throughout 'The Elephant Man', Treves simply calls him 'Merrick', as he no doubt did when he knew him, in line with the social conventions of the day. Only once does he mention a Christian name, and this is where he states that among the sparse information he obtained from the showman was the fact that 'his name was John Merrick'. At this point in the manuscript, hand-written in a fine calligraphy unusual if not unique in a member of the medical profession, Treves had originally put 'Joseph Merrick', then firmly crossed out 'Joseph' and corrected it to 'John'. The implication is unavoidable: Treves knew perfectly well that the Elephant Man's real name was Joseph and that he had misnamed him in his earlier papers. He therefore corrected it to keep the record straight and had no reason to dream that anyone would ever consider it further.

The publication of Treves's last book created many ripples of interest. It was widely reviewed in the specialist as well as the general press, and the journal known as the *World's Fair*, a publication devoted to news of interest to travelling showmen, carried an article on the Elephant Man culled from developed hip disease, which had left him permanently lame, so that he could only walk with a stick. He was thus denied all means of escape from his tormentors. As he told me later he could never run away. The other feature must be mentioned to emphasise his isolation from his kind. Although he was already repellent enough here arose from the bulbous skin-growth with which he was almost covered a very sickening stench which was hard to tolerate. From the showman I learnt nothing about the Elephant Man, except that he was English, that his name was John Merrick and that he was 21 years of age.

As at the time of my discovery of the Elephant Man I was the Lecturer on Anatomy at the Medical College opposite I was anxious to examine him in detail and to prepare an account of his abnormalities. I therefore arranged with the showman that I should interview his strange exhibit in my room at the College. I became at once conscious of a difficulty. The Elephant Man could not show himself in the streets. He would have been mobbed by the crowd and seized by the police. He was, in fact, as secluded from the world as the Man with the Iron Mask. He had, however, a disguise, although it was almost as startling as he was himself. It consisted of a long black cloak which reached to the ground. Whence the cloak had been obtained I cannot imagine. I had only seen such a garment on the stage wrapped about the figure of a Venetian bravo. The recluse was provided with a pair of bag-like slippers in which to hide his deformed feet. On his head was a cap of a kind that never before was seen. It was black like the cloak, had a wide peak and the general outline of a yachting cap. As the circumference of Merrick's head was that of a man's waist, the size of this head gear may be imagined. From the attachment of the peak a grey flannel curtain hung in front of the face. In this mask was cut a wide horizontal slit through which the wearer could look out. This costume, worn by a bent man hobbling along with a stick, is probably the most remarkable and the most uncanny that has as yet been designed. I arranged that Merrick should cross the road in a cab and to insure his immediate admission to the College I gave him my card. This card was destined to play a critical part in Merrick's life.

I made a careful examination of my visitor the result of which I embodied in a paper*. I made little of the man himself. He was shy, confused, not a little frightened

* British Medical Journal. Dec. 1886 and April 1890.

and evidently much cowed. Moreover his speech was almost unintelligible. The great bony mass that projected from his mouth blurred his utterance and made the articulation of certain words impossible. He returned in a cab to the place of exhibition and I assumed that I had seen the last of him, especially as I found next day that the show had been forbidden by the police and that the shop was empty.

Treves's material. It was this which came to the attention of Tom Norman, 'the Silver King', and stung him into writing a letter of injured pride in answer to the impression of him which Treves had put forward. Tom Norman had lived a life that was at times a precarious battle of wits, but he could fairly claim to have acted in his protégé's best interests. It was notable that Joseph himself could never be persuaded to talk disparagingly of the English showmen.

The letter to the *World's Fair* was incorporated by Tom Norman into the unpublished manuscript of the autobiography which he was putting together in his closing years. In this record of an artful and adventurous career, the Silver King, almost without realizing it, created the self-portrait of a man of remarkable courage, who knew his faults, could acknowledge failures, but continued to face the world with unconquered enthusiasm and grew to be illustrious in his profession. His triumphs included the mounting, during the First World War, of a great show in Trafalgar Square, London, in aid of war charities, and he earned his place in the fairground histories. To protect and promote the interests of his fellow showmen, he founded the Van Dwellers' Association, which later became the Showmen's Guild. Tom Norman's days, however, were also numbered. He was brought down by death at last after developing a throat tumour. He went out with a closing flourish, arguing good-naturedly with the surgeon over which of them was the better butcher. The ranks of the showmen, wrote the *Croydon Advertiser*, had lost a picturesque figure.

Of the other leading protagonists in the Elephant Man's story, Bishop Walsham How had died at the age of seventy-three during Queen Victoria's Diamond Jubilee year of 1897. As Bishop of Wakefield, he performed one last task of importance. A crisis had been precipitated when Sir Arthur Sullivan declined to set the words which the Poet Laureate, Alfred Austin, had written specially for the Jubilee service of thanksgiving in St Paul's Cathedral, saying that they were unworthy of his music. Bishop How was asked to step into the breach, and this he did, producing some alternative verses. In this way the bishop who had confirmed Joseph Merrick at the London Hospital also came to write Queen Victoria's Diamond Jubilee hymn:

> Thou has been mindful of Thine Own,
> And lo! we come confessing –
> 'Tis Thou has dowered our queenly throne
> With sixty years of blessing.

Plate 73 (opposite). In Treves's original manuscript of 'The Elephant Man', he clearly wrote 'Joseph' before making a deliberate mistake by correcting it to 'John'

Seven weeks after the celebrations, he died on holiday in western Ireland. His body was brought home to the Shropshire village of Whittington, where he had once officiated as parish priest, and there, respected for his integrity and obstinacy of purpose, the great churchman was buried, his grave marked by a simple stone slab.

At the beginning of that same Jubilee year, at 28 Justice Street, Leicester, on 30 January, Joseph Merrick's father, Joseph Rockley Merrick, died of chronic bronchitis. His death was registered, not by any member of his family, but by Mr George Preston, his next-door neighbour, who had been present at his passing. Of the Elephant Man's other relatives, we know only that his uncle, Charles Barnabus Merrick, continued to live in Leicester until his death in 1925. Joseph's little sister, Marion Eliza Merrick, unfortunately disappears entirely from view in the public records and we have no knowledge of her fate or destiny.

Sam Torr's daughter, Clara, who herself went on the halls, kept a diary in which she remembered how it had been at the Gaiety Palace of Varieties, Leicester, under her father's management.

Everything was going lovely as we thought.

We had a manager. He looked like a parson and knew about as much as one concerning the profession. We had several barmaids sometimes taking farthings for half-sovereigns.

We had several waiters always missing when they were wanted. One would be on the top flat roof waiting for the pill man to set his stall out. Then he would throw a bag of flour down and upset all the pills. Another waiter would be fastening the ends of the coat sleeves of the other waiters so that they couldn't get their arms through. We also had a chairman which they played all kinds of jokes on ...

But the crash came, all too soon. One morning my dear Mother came to me in terrible distress saying, 'Clara, everything will be sold in a few days and we shall be homeless. Whatever will become of us?'

'Don't grieve so, mother dear. Something will turn up!'

And something usually did turn up for Sam Torr, who was another true professional and who, it is said, made and lost three fortunes during the course of his life, through a cheerful mixture of generosity and profligacy. His London career was, however, finished by 1899, his style of presentation having by then gone more or less out of fashion. He went back to Leicester, but injured himself falling from the stage in 1904, while attempting to perform 'On the Back of Daddy-O' in a state of intoxication. He briefly became a publican, but sadly spent most of his declining years earning his

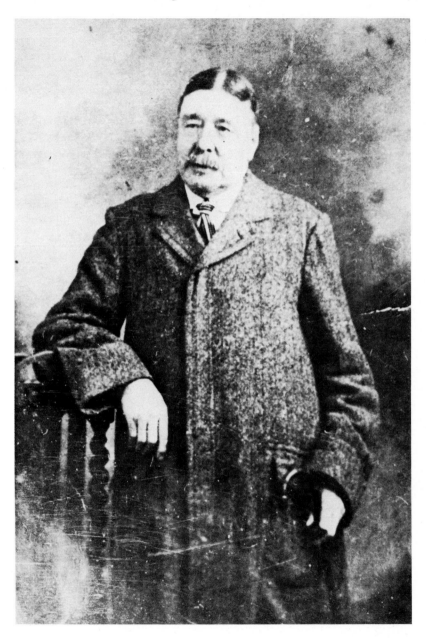

Plate 74. Sam Torr in his old age

bread and butter with a rather dubious turn performed in the back rooms of local hostelries. According to family recollection, he died quite gently in his own bed at the age of seventy-four, surrounded by those he loved. His end came in 1923, the same year as Treves's death and the publication of 'The Elephant Man'.

Madge Kendal retired from the stage in 1908, but lived on triumphantly as 'the matron of the British drama' until 1935, loaded down with honours and accolades, having received her DBE in 1926. She was, said Seymour Hicks, 'the very greatest of actresses'. 'No other English actress has such extraordinary skill,' wrote Ellen Terry, with whom Mrs Kendal was supposed to have enjoyed a life-long jealous rivalry, though like most such legends it was largely an invention of the press. On the other hand, Sir Cedric Hardwicke in *A Victorian in Orbit* had an altogether more waspish recollection of her.

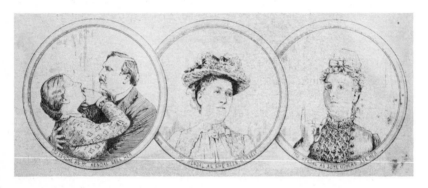

Plate 75. A cartoon makes satirical fun of Mrs Kendal, showing her (*left to right*) as Mr Kendal saw her, as she saw herself and as some others saw her

'She was one of a raft of sturdy, stage widows,' he wrote, 'whose sheer, awesome vitality had enabled them to outdistance their husbands in billings and longevity.' Being summoned to an audience with her after she had admired his creation of the role of King Magnus in Shaw's *The Apple Cart* turned out to be something of a trial, she making it clear 'that, in her view, the world had been running downhill since the death of dear Queen Victoria, accelerating with each year that passed'.

From the number of pressing invitations to return to her house, which followed the first encounter, I could appreciate that she was in dire need of company – and I could understand why. She reminded me forcibly of

Boadicea, that Amazonian English queen who mowed down Romans with her chariot wheels. Mrs Kendal was so terrifying that most contemporary members of our profession stayed clear in droves. Generally speaking, she regarded herself and her late husband as the last flowering of the dramatic arts.

Dr Reginald Tuckett, who first pressed Treves to go and view the Elephant Man, in 1893 went into a rural practice at Woodhouse Eaves, which lay close to the city of Leicester. He remained there as a general practitioner for more than fifty years, well known for his strength of personality and independence of viewpoint. He had refused to co-operate with Lloyd George's and Winston Churchill's National Insurance Act of 1911 when it was introduced, and the advent of Britain's National Health Service after the Second World War seemed to him to be the last straw. He finally retired in protest in 1948 at eighty-nine, dying two years later, one of the last of the impressive breed of physicians who were the products of the great teaching hospitals of Victorian London.

In the quiet hall of the Medical College of the London Hospital, in a glass case tucked away among other anatomical specimens in their glass cases, the skeleton of the Elephant Man stands, apparently ready to face up to the casual scrutiny of any passer-by. His surviving memorabilia are about him: the huge 'pillar-box' hat that Sam Roper had made for him and, at his feet, the cardboard model of the church which he put together and presented to Mrs Kendal. The plaster casts of his head and limbs that were made *post mortem* are also there, and perhaps convey something of the instinctive sense of shock and revulsion felt by so many when they first saw him. The skeleton itself, however, remains oddly touching, even moving, in its slightness of stature. The delicacy of the bones of the left arm still contrast strikingly with the random distortions of the bones on the opposite side of the body. The old hip injury can still be detected, and the curvature of the spine which accompanied the advance of the disease is also evident. On the skull, the effects are dramatic: the bone all down the right side of the head looks as though it has in some way been melted to the point where it began to run like a flow of lava.

Bedstead Square has been swept away by successive improvement and modernization schemes at the London Hospital, but the room which Joseph occupied in the basement still exists. Even this is not exactly as he knew it, since there has been some reorganization of the internal walls. It is now used as a storeroom. Large, asbestos-covered pipes from the hospital's central-heating system run around the walls, and it is impossible to conjure up any fragment of his presence. Perhaps it is only in our imaginations that he retains the power to haunt us.

Many of those who met and came to know Joseph Merrick were struck by his sensitive intelligence, by the sweetness of the personality beneath the horrifying outer shell. If there were elements of naïvety, this was inevitable in someone forced by circumstances to live so much of the 'normal' side of life inside his head and to take his experience of sophisticated living from books and romantic novels. Yet the lack of embitterment in his character had seemed a great puzzle, contrasting with the fierce cruelty of the attack which fate had launched on his physical body and the cruelties as abrasive which he had experienced at the hands of men.

In his earlier book on Merrick, *The Elephant Man: A Study in Human Dignity*, Ashley Montagu included an important chapter which explored this apparent contradiction in terms of Professor John Bowlby's seminal work on the effects on personality of maternal deprivation and, conversely, the importance of maternal love to a child if it is to develop into a socially healthy human being. Unfortunately, Professor Montagu had no choice but to draw his conclusions according to the face value of the information on Joseph's personal background which Frederick Treves happened to put into his essay. As the present book has shown, Treves actually succeeded in uncovering only the most fragmentary information about his patient's early life. The information on the period that he did include is also for the most part inaccurate or positively misleading.

Nevertheless Professor Montagu's final insights into the case match the facts as these emerge. He makes the point that if Merrick really had suffered the totally deprived life which Treves assumes, then the nature of his character would have been wholly beyond explanation. From the descriptions of Joseph's character, he deduces that he must have received a mother's loving care at least during the first few years of life, and that he must from time to time have subsequently been shown a degree of supportive kindness by others. It can now be confirmed that his mother's love was only withdrawn from him by her death when he was almost eleven, that after his father rejected him, his uncle, Charles Merrick, offered him support in so far as it was in his power, and that even the showmen who managed his exhibition in England, despite Treves's description of them as vampires, showed their concern for him in their own way.

Certain freaks have, in any case, demonstrated patience and good nature as integral parts of their characters. Perhaps there are also at times other compensatory processes at work. Tom Norman certainly claimed that all the freaks with whom he had had dealings were 'with but very few exceptions, as happy as the days are long, and were very contented with their lot in life'. At one time he had among his client showpieces the Scottish giantess, Mary Campbell,

> ... who used to sing 'Annie Laurie', and drank Scotch whisky and keep time with the next. But she was a dear old soul, good as gold. She lent me all her savings once, about £80, without asking, or a murmur. She was with me five years.

When William Hone interviewed M. Seurat, 'The Living Skeleton', in 1825 at the Chinese Saloon in Pall Mall, he found him neither unhappy nor miserable, despite the extreme emaciation of his frame. Seurat, in fact, had gone so far as to write a letter to the press in answer to an expression of moral indignation that had been sounded about his being put on show at all. His present situation was, he said, 'more happy than I ever yet enjoyed during my whole life, and is entirely conformable to my desires'. He had hopes that the proceeds of his exhibition would shortly allow him to return to France to live out his life at ease. As it turned out, poor Seurat was to die soon and leave his bones in London, where they went to join those of the Irish giant, Charles Byrne (also called O'Brien), and the Sicilian dwarf, Caroline Crachami, in the Hunterian Museum in the Royal College of Surgeons. With Seurat, however, it was the unembittered quality of his patience and gentleness that caught Hone's attention, and these clearly have parallels in the later example of Joseph Merrick.

The story of the Elephant Man and the Victorian surgeon, Frederick Treves, who took over the management of his destiny when every other path was closed, never ceases to show many facets and resonances. So long as it continues to catch hold of the imagination, then each generation will read into it its own mixtures of insight and prejudice. Like the relationships between Prospero and Caliban in Shakespeare's *The Tempest*, the emphases may seem to shift subtly in time, as new social parables are read in or drawn out. The monstrous whelp Caliban begins to shade into the figure of the Noble Savage, an ambiguous representation of man in a state of sexual innocence. The omnipotent magician Prospero, who can control the elements and hence the lives of men, is revealed to have feet of clay and to carry responsibility for the things which go wrong as well as those that can be put right. Interestingly enough, the fact that Treves tended to see Merrick, if only subconsciously, as a late manifestation of the Noble Savage is given away here and there by a piece of phrasing, as when he describes Joseph as 'an elemental being, so primitive' or 'this primitive creature'. Is it possible that

Treves was himself driven by that underlying sense of guilt which the doctor so often feels when he becomes aware of the fact that he must inevitably fail a certain patient when it comes to providing a cure?

It is perhaps one interpretation of the story to see Treves as a fundamentally exploiting figure sheltering behind an attitude of moral righteousness, while Merrick becomes the tame freak on whom society can safely lavish attention and so assuage its guilt at the vast inequalities of wealth created by the Industrial Revolution. This was a basis of interpretation which Bernard Pomerance used for his distinctive play *The Elephant Man* which enjoyed much success in its productions on the Broadway and London stages. But interpretation may imply a partial view of the facts, however valid or illuminating that view might be. The actual story of the Elephant Man seems constantly rich beyond the devices of fiction in its startling contrasts and turns of fate. The greatest presumption of all would be to think it ever possible to know or guess what it was truly like to have lived the life of Joseph Carey Merrick.

The closing and most valid image of Joseph which might be summoned up is that of a squat figure, extraordinary in outline, limping without hurry in the starlight across Bedstead Square and into the gardens of the London Hospital. The freedom to walk there unobserved and take the cool night air into his lungs, together with the scent of the spring flowers, became one with the hard-won freedom and dignity of his spirit under the stars: and so the limits to the span of his existence, the various griefs and injuries which his life sustained, even the hideousness of his flesh, were transformed eventually into matters of small importance.

APPENDIX ONE

The Autobiography of
Joseph Carey Merrick

I first saw the light on the 5th of August, 1860, I was born in Lee Street, Wharf Street, Leicester. The deformity which I am now exhibiting was caused by my mother being frightened by an Elephant; my mother was going along the street when a procession of Animals were passing by, there was a terrible crush of people to see them, and unfortunately she was pushed under the Elephant's feet, which frightened her very much; this occurring during a time of pregnancy was the cause of my deformity.

The measurement round my head is 36 inches, there is a large substance of flesh at the back as large as a breakfast cup, the other part in a manner of speaking is like hills and valleys, all lumped together, while the face is such a sight that no one could describe it. The right hand is almost the size and shape of an Elephant's fore-leg, measuring 12 inches round the wrist and 5 inches round one of the fingers; the other hand and arm is no larger than that of a girl ten years of age, although it is well proportioned. My feet and legs are covered with thick lumpy skin, also my body, like that of an Elephant, and almost the same colour, in fact, no one would believe until they saw it, that such a thing could exist. It was not perceived much at birth, but began to develop itself when at the age of 5 years.

I went to school like other children until I was about 11 or 12 years of age, when the greatest misfortune of my life occurred, namely – the death of my mother, peace to her, she was a good mother to me; after she died my father broke up his home and went to lodgings; unfortunately for me he married his landlady; henceforth I never had one moment's comfort, she having children of her own, and I not being so handsome as they, together with my deformity, she was the means of making my life a perfect misery; lame and deformed as I was, I ran, or rather walked away from home two or three times, but suppose father had some spark of parental feeling left, so he induced me to return home again. The best friend I had in those days was my father's brother, Mr Merrick, Hair Dresser, Church Gate, Leicester.

When about 13 years old, nothing would satisfy my stepmother until she got me out to work; I obtained employment at Messrs Freeman's, Cigar Manufacturers, and worked there about two years, but my right hand got too heavy for making cigars, so I had to leave them.

I was sent about the town to see if I could procure work, but being lame and deformed no one would employ me; when I went home for my meals, my step-mother used to say I had not been to seek for work. I was taunted and sneered at so that I would not go home to my meals, and used to stay in the streets with an hungry belly rather than return for anything to eat, what few half-meals I did have, I was taunted with the remark – 'That's more than you have earned.'

Being unable to get employment my father got me a pedlar's license to hawk the town, but being deformed, people would not come to the door to buy my wares. In consequence of my ill luck my life was again made a misery to me, so that I again ran away and went hawking on my own account, but my deformity had grown to such an extent, so that I could not move about the town without having a crowd of people gather round me. I then went into the infirmary at Leicester, where I remained for two or three years, when I had to undergo an operation on my face, having three or four ounces of flesh cut away; so thought I, I'll get my living by being exhibited about the country. Knowing Mr Sam Torr, Gladstone Vaults, Wharf Street, Leicester, went in for Novelties, I wrote to him, he came to see me, and soon arranged matters, recommending me to Mr Ellis, Bee-hive Inn, Nottingham, from whom I received the greatest kindness and attention.

In making my first appearance before the public, who have treated me well – in fact I may say I am as comfortable now as I was uncomfortable before. I must now bid my kind readers adieu.

> Was I so tall, could reach the pole,
>   Or grasp the ocean with a span;
> I would be measured by the soul,
>   The mind's the standard of the man.

APPENDIX TWO

The Elephant Man, amplified from an account published in the *British Medical Journal*

In November, 1886, a letter appeared in *The Times* from Mr Carr Gomm, chairman of the London Hospital, drawing attention to the sad case of Joseph Merrick. The letter attracted the notice of the charitable public, and through their very generous subscriptions the Hospital authorities were enabled to admit Merrick as a permanent inmate.

JOSEPH MERRICK is the subject of a very terrible congenital deformity, of so extreme a degree that he cannot venture into the streets, nor indeed into the garden of the Hospital. He cannot travel in any public conveyance nor mix with his fellow men. But for the kindness of his now numerous friends he would be cut off from all the common enjoyment of life.

Merrick is now about 27 years of age and was born of respectable parents in Leicester. Neither his father nor mother nor any of his relatives were in any way deformed. When quite a child his appearance was not sufficiently marked to attract any special attention, but by the time he had reached adult life the deformity of the face and limbs had attained to so extreme a degree that the unfortunate man was unable to follow any employment and physically prevented from learning any trade. His mother died when he was young, and his father, having married again, practically cast him off. There was nothing for him to do but to exhibit himself as a deformity in a penny show. Some features in the conformation of his head and limbs suggested the title of 'The Elephant Man', and as such Merrick was exhibited. He was dragged about from town to town and from fair to fair, and lived a life that was little better than a dismal slavery.

He was not treated with actual unkindness, but lived a life of almost solitary confinement, broken only when he appeared before a gaping and terrified audience as a hideous example of deformity.

Early in 1886 Mr Treves, one of the surgeons of the London Hospital, saw him as he was being exhibited in a room off the Whitechapel Road. The poor fellow was then crouching behind an old curtain endeavouring to warm himself over a brick which was heated by a gas jet. As soon as a sufficient number of pennies had been collected by the manager at the door, poor Merrick appeared in front of the curtain and exhibited himself in all his deformity. Merrick had a share in the proceeds of the exhibition, and by the exercise of great economy he had amassed nearly £50. The police, however, began to interfere and the exhibition was prohibited as against public decency. Unable to earn his livelihood by exhibiting himself any longer in England, he was persuaded to go over to Belgium, where he was taken in hand by an Austrian who acted as his manager. In Belgium, however, the exhibition was very soon prohibited by the police, and the miserable man and his manager were hunted from place to place. As soon as the Austrian saw that the exhibition was pretty well played out, he decamped with poor Merrick's very hardly saved capital of £50 and left him alone and absolutely destitute in a foreign country. Fortunately, however, he had something to pawn, by which he raised sufficient money to pay his passage back to England, for he felt that the only friend he had in the world was Mr Treves, of the London Hospital. He, therefore, though with much difficulty, made his way to London. At every station and landing place the curious crowd so thronged and dogged his steps that it was not an easy matter for him to get about. Indeed, at the quay great objections were raised to his being taken on board the steamer. When he reached the Hospital he had only the clothes in which he stood. For some time Merrick occupied a little ward in the attics, while every attempt was made to find him a permanent resting place. He had the greatest horror of the workhouse, and there seemed little to recommend the frequent suggestion that he should be placed in a blind asylum. The Royal Hospital for Incurables and the British Home for Incurables both declined to take him even if sufficient funds were forthcoming to pay for his maintenance for life. The subscription that was the result of Mr Carr Gomm's letter enabled the Hospital authorities to accept Merrick as a permanent resident. A room was built for him on the ground floor in a remote wing of the Institution. This room was comfortably furnished as a bedroom and sitting room, and to it was added a bathroom, for to Merrick a bath is not merely a luxury but, from the nature of his affliction, a daily necessity.

In this small room the elephant man spends his life, surrounded by innumerable tokens of the kindness of his friends. One of the first ladies to visit him, and certainly the first lady he had ever shaken hands with, was Mrs Maturin of Dublin. Mrs Kendal has been one of his kindest friends. She has supplied him with books, with pictures, with a musical box, and with numerous ornaments for his room, and had him taught basket-making as an amusement. He also owes to Mrs Kendal a very especial treat – a carefully planned and carefully disguised visit to a theatre.

Lady Knightley, in the summer of 1887, very kindly arranged a holiday for him, and with a little ingenuity Merrick found himself smuggled into a quiet cottage, in a remote part of the country far from the haunts of men, where he was made exceedingly happy.

The Hon. Mrs Gerald Wellesley became a frequent visitor, and gave him also a handsome musical box. Lady Dorothy Nevill presented him with a silver watch, of which he is very properly proud. Among his other kind friends may be mentioned the Hon. Mrs Jeune, to whom he indirectly owes his country holiday.

The great event in Merrick's life was a visit from T.R.H. the Prince and Princess of Wales and the Duke of Cambridge, in 1887. The Princess was exceedingly gracious, and not only did she give Merrick some flowers (most piously preserved), but she also sent him her photograph with her autograph attached. At the following Christmas Merrick was delighted to receive from Her Royal Highness three Christmas cards, with a kind message in the Princess' hand-writing on the back of each. Of the royal visit, of the portrait of the Princess, and of her Christmas cards, Merrick is never weary of talking.

The following abstract of the Medical Aspects of the case is obtained from Mr Treves' account published in the Pathological Society's Transactions, Vol. xxxvi, p. 494.

The elephant man is short, and lame through old disease of the left hip-joint. The deformity concerns the integuments and the bones. The subcutaneous tissue is greatly increased in amount in certain regions, with the result that the integument is raised prominently above the surrounding skin. This tissue is very loose, so that it can be raised from the deeper parts in great folds. In the right pectoral region, at the posterior aspect of the right axilla, and over the back, the affected skin forms heavy and remarkable pendulous flaps.

The skin is also subject to papillomatous growths, represented in some parts, as in the right clavicular region, by a mere roughening of the integument. Over the right side of the chest, the front of the abdomen, the back of the neck, and the right popliteal space, the growth is small; on the other hand, great masses of papillomata cover the back and the gluteal region. The eyelids, the ears, the entire left arm, nearly the whole of the front of the abdomen, the right and the left thigh, the left leg, and the back of the right leg, are free from disease.

The deformities of the osseous system are yet more remarkable. The cranial bones are deformed and overgrown, so that the circumference of the patient's head equals that of his waist. This deformity is better shown by the engravings than by any verbal description. Bony exostoses spring from the frontal bone, the posterior part of the parietals, and the occipital. Irregular elevations lie between these bosses, and all these deformities are very unsymmetrical. The right superior maxillary bone is greatly and irregularly enlarged. The right side of the hard palate and the right upper teeth occupy a lower level than the corresponding parts of the left side. The nose is turned to the left, and the lips are very prominent. The mouth cannot be shut.

All the bones of the right upper extremity, excepting the clavicle and scapula, and the bones of both feet, are enormously hypertrophied, without exostoses.

The patient prefers to sleep in a sitting posture with the head resting upon the knees.

The deformity is in no way allied to elephantiasis.

The following is added by Merrick himself.

'I should like to say a few words of thanks to all those that came forward with help and sympathy after my case was made known by Mr Carr Gomm in the public press. I have much to thank Mr Carr Gomm for, in letting me stay here, till something definite was done concerning me, as the London Hospital is not a place where patients are kept permanently, although the Committee have made arrangements for me to do so. I must also greatly thank the Hon. Mrs Wellesley, Mrs Kendal, and Lady Dorothy Nevill who have been very kind to me, and lastly my kind doctor, Mr Treves, whose visits I greatly prize, as many more in the hospital do, besides me. He is both friend and doctor to me. I have a nice bright room, made cheerful with flowers, books, and pictures. I am very comfortable, and I may say as happy as my condition will allow me to be.

> ' " 'Tis true my form is something odd,
>   But blaming me is blaming God;
>   Could I create myself anew
>   I would not fail in pleasing you.

' "If I could reach from pole to pole
Or grasp the ocean with a span,
I would be measured by the soul;
The mind's the standard of the man." ' '

APPENDIX THREE

'The Elephant Man'
by Sir Frederick Treves

In the Mile End Road, opposite to the London Hospital, there was (and possibly still is) a line of small shops. Among them was a vacant greengrocer's which was to let. The whole of the front of the shop, with the exception of the door, was hidden by a hanging sheet of canvas on which was the announcement that the Elephant Man was to be seen within and that the price of admission was twopence. Painted on the canvas in primitive colours was a life-size portrait of the Elephant Man. This very crude production depicted a frightful creature that could only have been possible in a nightmare. It was the figure of a man with the characteristics of an elephant. The transfiguration was not far advanced. There was still more of the man than of the beast. This fact – that it was still human – was the most repellent attribute of the creature. There was nothing about it of the pitiableness of the misshapened or the deformed, nothing of the grotesqueness of the freak, but merely the loathing insinuation of a man being changed into an animal. Some palm trees in the background of the picture suggested a jungle and might have led the imaginative to assume that it was in this wild that the perverted object had roamed.

When I first became aware of this phenomenon the exhibition was closed, but a well-informed boy sought the proprietor in a public house and I was granted a private view on payment of a shilling. The shop was empty and grey with dust. Some old tins and a few shrivelled potatoes occupied a shelf and some vague, vegetable refuse the window. The light in the place was dim, being obscured by the painted placard outside. The far end of the shop – where I expect the late proprietor sat at a desk – was cut off by a curtain or rather by a red tablecloth suspended from a cord by a few rings. The room was cold and dank, for it was the month of November. The year, I might say, was 1884.

The showman pulled back the curtain and revealed a bent figure crouching on a stool and covered by a brown blanket. In front of it, on a tripod, was a large brick heated by a Bunsen burner. Over this the creature was huddled to warm itself. It never moved when the curtain was drawn back. Locked up in an empty shop and lit by the faint blue light of the gas jet, this hunched-up figure was the embodiment of loneliness. It might have been a captive in a cavern or a wizard watching for unholy manifestations in the ghostly flame. Outside the sun was shining and one could hear the footsteps of the passers-by, a tune whistled by a boy and the commonplace hum of traffic in the road.

The showman – speaking as if to a dog – called out harshly: 'Stand up!' The thing arose slowly and let the blanket that covered its head and back fall to the ground. There stood revealed the most disgusting specimen of humanity that I have ever seen. In the course of my profession I had come upon lamentable deformities of the face due to injury or disease, as well as mutilations and contortions of the body depending upon like causes; but at no time had I met with such a degraded or perverted version of a human being as this lone figure displayed. He was naked to the waist, his feet were bare, he wore a pair of threadbare trousers that had once belonged to some fat gentleman's dress suit.

From the intensified painting in the street I had imagined the Elephant Man to be of gigantic size. This, however, was a little man below the average height and made to look shorter by the bowing of his back. The most striking feature about him was the enormous and misshapened head. From the brow there projected a huge bony mass like a loaf, while from the back of the head hung a bag of spongy, fungous-looking skin, the surface of which was comparable to brown cauliflower. On the top of the skull were a few long lank hairs. The osseous growth on the forehead almost occluded one eye. The circumference of the head was no less than that of the man's waist. From the upper jaw there projected another mass of bone. It protruded from the mouth like a pink stump, turning the upper lip inside out and making the mouth a mere slobbering aperture. This growth from the jaw had been so exaggerated in the painting as to appear to be a rudimentary trunk or tusk. The nose was merely a lump of flesh, only recognizable as a nose from its position. The face was no more capable of expression than a block of gnarled wood. The back was horrible, because from it hung, as far down as the middle of the thigh, huge, sack-like masses of flesh covered by the same loathsome cauliflower skin.

The right arm was of enormous size and shapeless. It suggested the limb of the subject of elephantiasis. It was overgrown also with pendent masses of the same cauliflower-like skin. The hand was large and clumsy – a fin or paddle rather than a hand. There was no distinction between the palm and the back. The thumb had the appearance of a radish, while the fingers might have been thick, tuberous roots. As a limb it was almost useless. The other arm was remarkable by contrast. It was not only normal but was, moreover, a delicately shaped limb covered with fine skin and provided with a beautiful hand which any woman might have envied. From the chest hung a bag of the same repulsive flesh. It was like a dewlap suspended from the neck of a lizard. The lower limbs had the characters of the deformed arm. They were unwieldy, dropsical looking and grossly misshapened.

To add a further burden to his trouble the wretched man, when a boy, developed hip disease, which had left him permanently lame, so that he could only walk with a stick. He was thus denied all means of escape from his tormentors. As he told me later, he could never run away. One other feature must be mentioned to emphasize his isolation from his kind. Although he was already repellent enough, there arose from the fungous skin-growth with which he was almost covered a very sickening stench which was hard to tolerate. From the showman I learnt nothing about the Elephant Man, except that he was English, that his name was John Merrick and that he was twenty-one years of age.

As at the time of my discovery of the Elephant Man I was the Lecturer on Anatomy at the Medical College opposite, I was anxious to examine him in detail and to prepare an account of his abnormalities. I therefore arranged with the showman that I should interview his strange exhibit in my room at the college. I became at once conscious of a difficulty. The Elephant Man could not show himself in the streets. He would have been mobbed by the crowd and seized by the police. He was, in fact, as secluded from the world as the Man with the Iron Mask. He had, however, a disguise, although it was almost as startling as he was himself. It consisted of a long black cloak which reached to the ground. Whence the cloak had been obtained I cannot imagine. I had only seen such a garment on the stage wrapped about the figure of a Venetian bravo. The recluse was provided with a pair of bag-like slippers in which to hide his deformed feet. On his head was a cap of a kind that never before was seen. It was black like the cloak, had a wide peak, and the general outline of a yachting cap. As the circumference of Merrick's head was that of a man's waist, the size of this head-gear may be imagined. From the attachment of the peak a grey flannel curtain hung in front of the face. In this mask was cut a wide horizontal slit through which the wearer could look out. This costume, worn by a bent man hobbling along with a stick, is probably the most remarkable and the most uncanny that has as yet been designed. I arranged that Merrick should cross the road in a cab, and to insure his immediate admission to the college I gave him my card. This card was destined to play a critical part in Merrick's life.

I made a careful examination of my visitor the result of which I embodied in a paper.[1] I made little of the man himself. He was shy, confused, not a little frightened and evidently much cowed. Moreover, his speech was almost unintelligible. The great bony mass that projected from his mouth blurred his utterance and made the articulation of certain words impossible. He returned in a cab to the place of exhibition, and I assumed that I had seen the last of him, especially as I found next day that the show had been forbidden by the police and that the shop was empty.

I supposed that Merrick was imbecile and had been imbecile from birth. The fact that his face was incapable of expression, that his speech was a mere spluttering and his attitude that of one whose mind was void of all emotions and concerns gave grounds for this belief. The conviction was no doubt encouraged by the hope that his intellect was the blank I imagined it to be. That he could appreciate his position was unthinkable. Here was a man in the heyday of youth who was so vilely deformed that everyone he met confronted him with a look of horror and disgust. He was taken about the country to be exhibited as a monstrosity and an object of loathing. He was shunned like a leper, housed like a wild beast, and got his only view of the world from a peephole in a showman's cart. He was, moreover, lame, had but one available arm, and could hardly make his utterances understood. It was not until I came to know that Merrick was highly intelligent, that he possessed an acute sensibility and – worse than all – a romantic imagination that I realized the overwhelming tragedy of his life.

The episode of the Elephant Man was, I imagined, closed; but I was fated to meet him again – two years later – under more dramatic conditions. In England the showman and Merrick had been moved on from place to place by the police, who considered the exhibition degrading and among the things that could not be allowed. It was hoped that in the uncritical retreats of Mile End a more abiding peace would be found. But it was not to be. The official mind there, as elsewhere, very properly decreed that the public exposure of Merrick and his deformities transgressed the limits of decency. The show must close.

The showman, in despair, fled with his charge to the Continent. Whither he roamed at first I do not know; but he came finally to Brussels. His

---

1 *British Medical Journal*, Dec. 1886, and April 1890

reception was discouraging. Brussels was firm; the exhibition was banned; it was brutal, indecent and immoral, and could not be permitted within the confines of Belgium. Merrick was thus no longer of value. He was no longer a source of profitable entertainment. He was a burden. He must be got rid of. The elimination of Merrick was a simple matter. He could offer no resistance. He was as docile as a sick sheep. The impresario, having robbed Merrick of his paltry savings, gave him a ticket to London, saw him into the train and no doubt in parting condemned him to perdition.

His destination was Liverpool Street. The journey may be imagined. Merrick was in his alarming outdoor garb. He would be harried by an eager mob as he hobbled along the quay. They would run ahead to get a look at him. They would lift the hem of his cloak to peep at his body. He would try to hide in the train or in some dark corner of the boat, but never could he be free from that ring of curious eyes or from those whispers of fright and aversion. He had but a few shillings in his pocket and nothing either to eat or drink on the way. A panic-dazed dog with a label on his collar would have received some sympathy and possibly some kindness. Merrick received none.

What was he to do when he reached London? He had not a friend in the world. He knew no more of London than he knew of Pekin. How could he find a lodging, or what lodging-house keeper would dream of taking him in? All he wanted was to hide. What most he dreaded were the open street and the gaze of his fellow-men. If even he crept into a cellar the horrid eyes and the still more dreaded whispers would follow him to its depths. Was there ever such a home-coming!

At Liverpool Street he was rescued from the crowd by the police and taken into the third-class waiting-room. Here he sank on the floor in the darkest corner. The police were at a loss what to do with him. They had dealt with strange and mouldy tramps, but never with such an object as this. He could not explain himself. His speech was so maimed that he might as well have spoken in Arabic. He had, however, something with him which he produced with a ray of hope. It was my card.

The card simplified matters. It made it evident that this curious creature had an acquaintance and that the individual must be sent for. A messenger was dispatched to the London Hospital which is comparatively near at hand. Fortunately I was in the building and returned at once with the messenger to the station. In the waiting-room I had some difficulty in making a way through the crowd, but there, on the floor in the corner, was Merrick. He looked a mere heap. It seemed as if he had been thrown there like a bundle. He was so huddled up and so helpless looking that he might have had both his arms and his legs broken. He seemed pleased to see me, but he was nearly done. The journey and want of food had reduced him to the last stage of exhaustion. The police kindly helped him into a cab, and I drove him at once to the hospital. He appeared to be content, for he fell asleep almost as soon as he was seated and slept to the journey's end. He never said a word, but seemed to be satisfied that all was well.

In the attics of the hospital was an isolation ward with a single bed. It was used for emergency purposes – for a case of delirium tremens, for a man who had become suddenly insane or for a patient with an undetermined fever. Here the Elephant Man was deposited on a bed, was made comfortable and was supplied with food. I had been guilty of an irregularity in admitting such a case, for the hospital was neither a refuge nor a home for incurables. Chronic cases were not accepted, but only those requiring active treatment, and Merrick was not in need of such treatment. I applied to the sympathetic chairman of the committee, Mr Carr Gomm, who not only was good enough to approve my action but who agreed with me that Merrick must not again be turned out into the world.

Mr Carr Gomm wrote a letter to *The Times* detailing the circumstances of the refugee and asking for money for his support. So generous is the English public that in a few days – I think in a week – enough money was forthcoming to maintain Merrick for life without any charge upon the hospital funds. There chanced to be two empty rooms at the back of the hospital which were little used. They were on the ground floor, were out of the way, and opened upon a large courtyard called Bedstead Square, because here the iron beds were marshalled for cleaning and painting. The front room was converted into a bed-sitting room and the smaller chamber into a bathroom. The condition of Merrick's skin rendered a bath at least once a day a necessity, and I might here mention that with the use of the bath the unpleasant odour to which I have referred ceased to be noticeable. Merrick took up his abode in the hospital in December, 1886.

Merrick had now something he had never dreamed of, never supposed to be possible – a home of his own for life. I at once began to make myself acquainted with him to endeavour to understand his mentality. It was a study of much interest. I very soon learnt his speech so that I could talk freely with him. This afforded him great satisfaction, for, curiously enough, he had a passion for conversation, yet all his life had had no one to talk to. I – having then much leisure – saw him almost every day, and made a point of spending some two hours with him every Sunday morning when he would chatter almost without ceasing. It was unreasonable to expect one nurse to attend to him continuously, but there was no lack of temporary volunteers. As they did not all acquire his speech it came about that I had occasionally to act as an interpreter.

I found Merrick, as I have said, remarkably intelligent. He had learnt to read and had become a most voracious reader. I think he had been taught when he was in hospital with his diseased hip. His range of books was limited. The Bible and Prayer Book he knew intimately, but he had subsisted for the most part upon newspapers, or rather upon such fragments of old journals as he had chanced to pick up. He had read a few stories and some elementary lesson books, but the delight of his life was a romance, especially a love romance. These tales were very real to him, as real as any narrative in the Bible, so that he would tell them to me as incidents in the lives of people who had lived. In his outlook upon the world he was a child, yet a child with some of the tempestuous feelings of a man. He was an elemental being, so primitive that he might have spent the twenty-three years of his life immured in a cave.

Of his early days I could learn but little. He was very loath to talk about the past. It was a nightmare, the shudder of which was still upon him. He was born, he believed, in or about Leicester. Of his father he knew absolutely nothing. Of his mother he had some memory. It was very faint and had, I think, been elaborated in his mind into something definite. Mothers figured in the tales he had read, and he wanted his mother to be one of those comfortable lullaby-singing persons who are so lovable. In his subconscious mind there was apparently a germ of recollection in which someone figured who had been kind to him. He clung to this conception and made it more real by invention, for since the day when he could toddle no one had been kind to him. As an infant he must have been repellent, although his deformities did not become gross until he had attained his full stature.

It was a favourite belief of his that his mother was beautiful. The fiction was, I am aware, one of his own making, but it was a great joy to him. His mother, lovely as she may have been, basely deserted him when he was very small, so small that his earliest clear memories were of the workhouse to which he had been taken. Worthless and inhuman as this mother was, he spoke of her with pride and even with reverence. Once, when referring to his own appearance, he said: 'It *is* very strange, for, you see, mother was so beautiful.'

The rest of Merrick's life up to the time that I met him at Liverpool Street Station was one dull record of degradation and squalor. He was dragged from town to town and from fair to fair as if he were a strange beast in a cage. A dozen times a day he would have to expose his nakedness and his piteous deformities before a gaping crowd who greeted him with such mutterings as 'Oh! what a horror! What a beast!' He had had no childhood. He had had no boyhood. He had never experienced pleasure. He knew nothing of the joy of living nor of the fun of things. His sole idea of happiness was to creep into the dark and hide. Shut up alone in a booth, awaiting the next exhibition, how mocking must have sounded the laughter and merriment of the boys and girls outside who were enjoying the 'fun of the fair'! He had no past to look back upon and no future to look forward to. At the age of twenty he was a creature without hope. There was nothing in front of him but a vista of caravans creeping along a road, of rows of glaring show tents and of circles of staring eyes with, at the end, the spectacle of a broken man in a poor law infirmary.

Those who are interested in the evolution of character might speculate as to the effect of this brutish life upon a sensitive and intelligent man. It would be reasonable to surmise that he would become a spiteful and malignant misanthrope, swollen with venom and filled with hatred of his fellow-men, or, on the other hand, that he would degenerate into a despairing melancholic on the verge of idiocy. Merrick, however, was no such being. He had passed through the fire and had come out unscathed. His troubles had ennobled him. He showed himself to be a gentle, affectionate and lovable creature, as amiable as a happy woman, free from any trace of cynicism or resentment, without a grievance and without an unkind word for anyone. I have never heard him complain. I have never heard him deplore his ruined life or resent the treatment he had received at the hands of callous keepers. His journey through life had been indeed along a *via dolorosa*, the road had been uphill all the way, and now, when the night was at its blackest and the way most steep, he had suddenly found himself, as it were, in a friendly inn, bright with light and warm with welcome. His gratitude to those about him was pathetic in its sincerity and eloquent in the childlike simplicity with which it was expressed.

As I learnt more of this primitive creature I found that there were two anxieties which were prominent in his mind and which he revealed to me with diffidence. He was in the occupation of the rooms assigned to him and had been assured that he would be cared for to the end of his days. This, however, he found hard to realize, for he often asked me timidly to what place he would next be moved. To understand his attitude it is necessary to remember that he had been moving on and moving on all his life. He knew no other state of existence. To him it was normal. He had passed from the workhouse to the hospital, from the hospital back to the workhouse, then from this town to that town or from one showman's caravan to another. He had never known a home nor any semblance of one. He had no possessions.

His sole belongings, besides his clothes and some books, were the monstrous cap and the cloak. He was a wanderer, a pariah and an outcast. That his quarters at the hospital were his for life he could not understand. He could not rid his mind of the anxiety which had pursued him for so many years – where am I to be taken next?

Another trouble was his dread of his fellow-men, his fear of people's eyes, the dread of being always stared at, the lash of the cruel mutterings of the crowd. In his home in Bedstead Square he was secluded; but now and then a thoughtless porter or a wardmaid would open his door to let curious friends have a peep at the Elephant Man. It therefore seemed to him as if the gaze of the world followed him still.

Influenced by these two obsessions he became, during his first few weeks at the hospital, curiously uneasy. At last, with much hesitation, he said to me one day: 'When I am next moved can I go to a blind asylum or to a lighthouse?' He had read about blind asylums in the newspapers and was attracted by the thought of being among people who could not see. The lighthouse had another charm. It meant seclusion from the curious. There at least no one could open a door and peep in at him. Then he would forget that he had once been the Elephant Man. There he would escape the vampire showman. He had never seen a lighthouse, but he had come upon a picture of the Eddystone, and it appeared to him that this lonely column of stone in the waste of the sea was such a home as he had longed for.

I had no great difficulty in ridding Merrick's mind of these ideas. I wanted him to get accustomed to his fellow-men, to become a human being himself and to be admitted to the communion of his kind. He appeared day by day less frightened, less haunted looking, less anxious to hide, less alarmed when he saw his door being opened. He got to know most of the people about the place, to be accustomed to their comings and goings, and to realize that they took no more than a friendly notice of him. He could only go out after dark, and on fine nights ventured to take a walk in Bedstead Square clad in his black cloak and his cap. His greatest adventure was on one moonless evening when he walked alone as far as the hospital garden and back again.

To secure Merrick's recovery and to bring him, as it were, to life once more, it was necessary that he should make the acquaintance of men and women who would treat him as a normal and intelligent young man and not as a monster of deformity. Women I felt to be more important than men in bringing about his transformation. Women were the more frightened of him, the more disgusted at his appearance and the more apt to give way to irrepressible expressions of aversion when they came into his presence. Moreover, Merrick had an admiration of women of such a kind that it attained almost to adoration. This was not the outcome of his personal experience. They were not real women but the products of his imagination. Among them was the beautiful mother surrounded, at a respectful distance, by heroines from the many romances he had read.

His first entry to the hospital was attended by a regrettable incident. He had been placed on the bed in the little attic, and a nurse had been instructed to bring him some food. Unfortunately she had not been fully informed of Merrick's unusual appearance. As she entered the room she saw on the bed, propped up by white pillows, a monstrous figure as hideous as an Indian idol. She at once dropped the tray she was carrying and fled, with a shriek, through the door. Merrick was too weak to notice much, but the experience, I am afraid, was not new to him.

He was looked after by volunteer nurses whose ministrations were somewhat formal and constrained. Merrick, no doubt, was conscious that their service was purely official, that they were merely doing what they were told to do and that they were acting rather as automata than as women. They did not help him to feel that he was of their kind. On the contrary they, without knowing it, made him aware that the gulf of separation was immeasurable.

Feeling this, I asked a friend of mine, a young and pretty widow, if she thought she could enter Merrick's room with a smile, wish him good morning and shake him by the hand. She said she could and she did. The effect upon poor Merrick was not quite what I had expected. As he let go her hand he bent his head on his knees and sobbed until I thought he would never cease. The interview was over. He told me afterwards that this was the first woman who had ever smiled at him, and the first woman, in the whole of his life, who had shaken hands with him. From this day the transformation of Merrick commenced and he began to change, little by little, from a hunted thing into a man. It was a wonderful change to witness and one that never ceased to fascinate me.

Merrick's case attracted much attention in the papers, with the result that he had a constant succession of visitors. Everybody wanted to see him. He must have been visited by almost every lady of note in the social world. They were all good enough to welcome him with a smile and to shake hands with him. The Merrick whom I had found shivering behind a rag of a curtain in an empty shop was now conversant with duchesses and countesses and other ladies of high degree. They brought him presents, made his room bright with ornaments and pictures, and, what pleased him more than all, supplied him with books. He soon had a large library and most of his day was spent in reading. He was not the least spoiled; not the least puffed up; he never asked for anything; never presumed upon the kindness meted out to him, and was always humbly and profoundly grateful. Above all he lost his shyness. He liked to see his door pushed upon and people look in. He became acquainted with most of the frequenters of Bedstead Square, would chat with them at his window and show them some of his choicest presents. He improved in his speech, although to the end his utterances were not easy for strangers to understand. He was beginning, moreover, to be less conscious of his unsightliness, a little disposed to think it was, after all, not so very extreme. Possibly this was aided by the circumstance that I would not allow a mirror of any kind in his room.

The height of his social development was reached on an eventful day when Queen Alexandra – then Princess of Wales – came to the hospital to pay him a special visit. With that kindness which marked every act of her life, the Queen entered Merrick's room smiling and shook him warmly by the hand. Merrick was transported with delight. This was beyond even his most extravagant dream. The Queen made many people happy, but I think no gracious act of hers ever caused such happiness as she brought into Merrick's room when she sat by his chair and talked to him as to a person she was glad to see.

Merrick, I may say, was now one of the most contented creatures I have chanced to meet. More than once he said to me: 'I am happy every hour of the day.' This was good to think upon when I recalled the half-dead heap of miserable humanity I had seen in the corner of the waiting-room at Liverpool Street. Most men of Merrick's age would have expressed their joy and sense of contentment by singing or whistling when they were alone. Unfortunately poor Merrick's mouth was so deformed that he could neither whistle nor sing. He was satisfied to express himself by beating time upon the pillow to some tune that was ringing in his head. I have many times found him so occupied when I have entered his room unexpectedly. One thing that always struck me as sad about Merrick was the fact that he could not smile. Whatever his delight might be, his face remained expressionless. He could weep but he could not smile.

The Queen paid Merrick many visits and sent him every year a Christmas card with a message in her own handwriting. On one occasion she sent him a signed photograph of herself. Merrick, quite overcome, regarded it as a sacred object and would hardly allow me to touch it. He cried over it, and after it was framed had it put up in his room as a kind of ikon. I told him that he must write to Her Royal Highness to thank her for her goodness. This he was pleased to do, as he was very fond of writing letters, never before in his life having had anyone to write to. I allowed the letter to be dispatched unedited. It began 'My dear Princess' and ended 'Yours very sincerely'.

Unorthodox as it was it was expressed in terms any courtier would have envied.

Other ladies followed the Queen's gracious example and sent their photographs to this delighted creature who had been all his life despised and rejected of men. His mantelpiece and table became so covered with photographs of handsome ladies, with dainty knicknacks and pretty trifles that they may almost have befitted the apartment of an Adonis-like actor or of a famous tenor.

Through all these bewildering incidents and through the glamour of this great change Merrick still remained in many ways a mere child. He had all the invention of an imaginative boy or girl, the same love of 'make-believe', the same instinct of 'dressing up' and of personating heroic and impressive characters. This attitude of mind was illustrated by the following incident. Benevolent visitors had given me, from time to time, sums of money to be expended for the comfort of the *ci-devant* Elephant Man. When one Christmas was approaching I asked Merrick what he would like me to purchase as a Christmas present. He rather startled me by saying shyly that he would like a dressing-bag with silver fittings. He had seen a picture of such an article in an advertisement which he had furtively preserved.

The association of a silver-fitted dressing-bag with the poor wretch wrapped up in a dirty blanket in an empty shop was hard to comprehend. I fathomed the mystery in time, for Merrick made little secret of the fancies that haunted his boyish brain. Just as a small girl with a tinsel coronet and a window curtain for a train will realize the conception of a countess on her way to court, so Merrick loved to imagine himself a dandy and a young man about town. Mentally, no doubt, he had frequently 'dressed up' for the part. He could 'make-believe' with great effect, but he wanted something to render his fancied character more realistic. Hence the jaunty bag which was to assume the function of the toy coronet and the window curtain that could transform a mite with a pigtail into a countess.

As a theatrical 'property' the dressing-bag was ingenious, since there was little else to give substance to the transformation. Merrick could not wear the silk hat of the dandy nor, indeed, any kind of hat. He could not adapt his body to the trimly cut coat. His deformity was such that he could wear neither collar nor tie, while in association with his bulbous feet the young blood's patent leather shoe was unthinkable. What was there left to make up the character? A lady had given him a ring to wear on his undeformed hand, and a noble lord had presented him with a very stylish walking-stick. But these things, helpful as they were, were hardly sufficing.

The dressing-bag, however, was distinctive, was explanatory and entirely characteristic. So the bag was obtained and Merrick the Elephant Man became in the seclusion of his chamber, the Piccadilly exquisite, the young spark, the gallant, the 'nut'. When I purchased the article I realized that as Merrick could never travel he could hardly want a dressing-bag. He could not use the silver-backed brushes and the comb because he had no hair to brush. The ivory-handled razors were useless because he could not shave. The deformity of his mouth rendered an ordinary toothbrush of no avail, and as his monstrous lips could not hold a cigarette the cigarette-case was a mockery. The silver shoe-horn would be of no service in the putting on of his ungainly slippers, while the hat-brush was quite unsuited to the peaked cap with its visor.

Still the bag was an emblem of the real swell and of the knockabout Don Juan of whom he had read. So every day Merrick laid out upon his table, with proud precision, the silver brushes, the razors, the shoe-horn and the silver cigarette-case which I had taken care to fill with cigarettes. The contemplation of these gave him great pleasure, and such is the power of self-deception that they convinced him he was the 'real thing'.

I think there was just one shadow in Merrick's life. As I have already said, he had a lively imagination; he was romantic; he cherished an emotional regard for women and his favourite pursuit was the reading of love stories. He fell in love – in a humble and devotional way – with, I think, every attractive lady he saw. He, no doubt, pictured himself the hero of many a passionate incident. His bodily deformity had left unmarred the instincts and feelings of his years. He was amorous. He would like to have been a lover, to have walked with the beloved object in the languorous shades of some beautiful garden and to have poured into her ear all the glowing utterances that he had rehearsed in his heart. And yet – the pity of it! – imagine the feelings of such a youth when he saw nothing but a look of horror creep over the face of every girl whose eyes met his. I fancy when he talked of life among the blind there was a half-formed idea in his mind that he might be able to win the affection of a woman if only she were without eyes to see.

As Merrick developed he began to display certain modest ambitions in the direction of improving his mind and enlarging his knowledge of the world. He was as curious as a child and as eager to learn. There were so many things he wanted to know and see. In the first place he was anxious to view the interior of what he called 'a real house', such a house as figured in many of the tales he knew, a house with a hall, a drawing-room where guests were received and a dining-room with plate on the sideboard and with easy chairs into which the hero could 'fling himself'. The workhouse, the common lodging-house and a variety of mean garrets were all the residences he knew.

To satisfy this wish I drove him up to my small house in Wimpole Street. He was absurdly interested and examined everything in detail and with untiring curiosity. I could not show him the pampered menials and the powdered footmen of whom he had read, nor could I produce the white marble staircase of the mansion of romance nor the gilded mirrors and the brocaded divans which belong to that style of residence. I explained that the house was a modest dwelling of the Jane Austen type, and as he had read *Emma* he was content.

A more burning ambition of his was to go to the theatre. It was a project very difficult to satisfy. A popular pantomime was then in progress at Drury Lane Theatre, but the problem was how so conspicuous a being as the Elephant Man could get there, and how he was to see the performance without attracting the notice of the audience and causing a panic or, at least, an unpleasant diversion. The whole matter was most ingeniously carried through by that kindest of women and most able of actresses – Mrs Kendal. She made the necessary arrangements with the lessee of the theatre. A box was obtained. Merrick was brought up in a carriage with drawn blinds and was allowed to make use of the royal entrance so as to reach the box by a private stair. I had begged three of the hospital sisters to don evening dress and to sit in the front row in order to 'dress' the box, on the one hand, and to form a screen for Merrick on the other. Merrick and I occupied the back of the box which was kept in shadow. All went well, and no one saw a figure, more monstrous than any on the stage, mount the staircase or cross the corridor.

One has often witnessed the unconstrained delight of a child at its first pantomime, but Merrick's rapture was much more intense as well as much more solemn. Here was a being with the brain of a man, the fancies of a youth and the imagination of a child. His attitude was not so much that of delight as of wonder and amazement. He was awed. He was enthralled. The spectacle left him speechless, so that if he were spoken to he took no heed. He often seemed to be panting for breath. I could not help comparing him with a man of his own age in the stalls. This satiated individual was bored to distraction, would look wearily at the stage from time to time and then yawn as if he had not slept for nights; while at the same time Merrick was thrilled by a vision that was almost beyond his comprehension. Merrick talked of this pantomime for weeks and weeks. To him, as to a child with the faculty of make-believe, everything was real; the palace was the home of kings, the princess was of royal blood, the fairies were as undoubted as the children in the street, while the dishes at the banquet were of unquestionable gold. He did not like to discuss it as a play but rather as a vision of some actual world.

When this mood possessed him he would say: 'I wonder what the prince did after we left,' or 'Do you think that poor man is still in the dungeon?' and so on and so on.

The splendour and display impressed him, but, I think, the ladies of the ballet took a still greater hold upon his fancy. He did not like the ogres and the giants, while the funny men impressed him as irreverent. Having no experience as a boy of romping and ragging, of practical jokes or of 'larks', he had little sympathy with the doings of the clown, but, I think (moved by some mischievous instinct in his subconscious mind), he was pleased when the policeman was smacked in the face, knocked down and generally rendered undignified.

Later on another longing stirred the depths of Merrick's mind. It was a desire to see the country, a desire to live in some green secluded spot and there learn something about flowers and the ways of animals and birds. The country as viewed from a wagon on a dusty high road was all the country he knew. He had never wandered among the fields nor followed the windings of a wood. He had never climbed to the brow of a breezy down. He had never gathered flowers in a meadow. Since so much of his reading dealt with country life he was possessed by the wish to see the wonders of that life himself.

This involved a difficulty greater than that presented by a visit to the theatre. The project was, however, made possible on this occasion also by the kindness and generosity of a lady – Lady Knightley – who offered Merrick a holiday home in a cottage on her estate. Merrick was conveyed to the railway station in the usual way, but as he could hardly venture to appear on the platform the railway authorities were good enough to run a second-class carriage into a distant siding. To this point Merrick was driven and was placed in the carriage unobserved. The carriage, with the curtains drawn, was then attached to the mainline train.

He duly arrived at the cottage, but the housewife (like the nurse at the hospital) had not been made clearly aware of the unfortunate man's appearance. Thus it happened that when Merrick presented himself his hostess, throwing her apron over her head, fled, gasping, to the fields. She affirmed that such a guest was beyond her powers of endurance for, when she saw him, she was 'that took' as to be in danger of being permanently 'all of a tremble'.

Merrick was then conveyed to a gamekeeper's cottage which was hidden from view and was close to the margin of a wood. The man and his wife were able to tolerate his presence. They treated him with the greatest kindness, and with them he spent the one supreme holiday of his life. He could roam where he pleased. He met no one on his wanderings, for the wood was preserved and denied to all but the gamekeeper and the forester.

There is no doubt that Merrick passed in this retreat the happiest time he had as yet experienced. He was alone in a land of wonders. The breath of the country passed over him like a healing wind. Into the silence of the wood the fearsome voice of the showman could never penetrate. No cruel eyes could peep at him through the friendly undergrowth. It seemed as if in this place of peace all stain had been wiped away from his sullied past. The Merrick who had once crouched terrified in the filthy shadows of a Mile End shop was now sitting in the sun, in a clearing among the trees, arranging a bunch of violets he had gathered.

His letters to me were the letters of a delighted and enthusiastic child. He gave an account of his trivial adventures, of the amazing things he had seen, and of the beautiful sounds he had heard. He had met with strange birds, had startled a hare from her form, had made friends with a fierce dog, and had watched the trout darting in a stream. He sent me some of the wild flowers he had picked. They were of the commonest and most familiar kind, but they were evidently regarded by him as rare and precious specimens.

He came back to London, to his quarters in Bedstead Square, much improved in health, pleased to be 'home' again and to be once more among his books, his treasures and his many friends.

Some six months after Merrick's return from the country he was found dead in bed. This was in April, 1890. He was lying on his back as if asleep, and had evidently died suddenly and without a struggle, since not even the coverlet of the bed was disturbed. The method of his death was peculiar. So large and so heavy was his head that he could not sleep lying down. When he assumed the recumbent position the massive skull was inclined to drop backwards, with the result that he experienced no little distress. The attitude he was compelled to assume when he slept was very strange. He sat up in bed with his back supported by pillows, his knees were drawn up, and his arms clasped round his legs, while his head rested on the points of his bent knees.

He often said to me that he wished he could lie down to sleep 'like other people'. I think on this last night he must, with some determination, have made the experiment. The pillow was soft, and the head, when placed on it, must have fallen backwards and caused a dislocation of the neck. Thus it came about that his death was due to the desire that had dominated his life – the pathetic but hopeless desire to be 'like other people'.

As a specimen of humanity, Merrick was ignoble and repulsive; but the spirit of Merrick, if it could be seen in the form of the living, would assume the figure of an upstanding and heroic man, smooth browed and clean of limb, and with eyes that flashed undaunted courage.

His tortured journey had come to an end. All the way he, like another, had borne on his back a burden almost too grievous to bear. He had been plunged into the Slough of Despond, but with manly steps had gained the farther shore. He had been made 'a spectacle to all men' in the heartless streets of the Vanity Fair. He had been ill-treated and reviled and bespattered with the mud of Disdain. He had escaped the clutches of the Giant Despair, and at last had reached the 'Place of Deliverance', where 'his burden loosed from off his shoulders and fell from off his back, so that he saw it no more.'

BIBLIOGRAPHY

1. BOOKS AND ARTICLES DIRECTLY RELEVANT TO THE STORY
OF THE ELEPHANT MAN OR HIS CLINICAL CONDITION

Battiscombe, Georgina, *Queen Alexandra*, Constable, London, 1969.

Bland-Sutton, Sir John, *The Story of a Surgeon*, Methuen, London, 1930.

Boyd, William, *Textbook of Pathology*, Henry Kimpton, London, 1947.

Brain, Russell, *Diseases of the Nervous System*, 5th edition, Oxford University Press, 1956.

Brasfield, Richard D., and Gupta, Tapas K. Das, 'Von Recklinghausen's Disease: A Clinicopathological Study', *Annals of Surgery*, vol. 175, no. 1, January 1972, pp. 86-104.

Cambridge, 2nd Duke of, *George, Duke of Cambridge: A Memoir of His Private Life, Based on the Journals and Correspondence of H.R.H.*, ed. J.E. Shepherd, 2 vols., Longman, London, 1906.

Carswell, Heather, 'Elephant Man Had More Than Neurofibromatosis', *Journal of the American Medical Association*, vol. 248, no. 9, 3 September 1982, pp. 1032-3; based on *Seminars of Roentgenology*, vol. 17, 1982, p. 153.

Clarke-Kennedy, A.E., *The London: A Study of the Voluntary Hospital System*, vol. 2: *The Second Hundred Years, 1840-1948*, Pitman Medical Publishing, London, 1963.

Crocker, H. Radcliffe, *Diseases of the Skin: a Review of 51,000 Cases of Skin Disorder*, 3rd edition, vol. 2, Lewis, London, 1905.

Crowe, F.W., Schull, W.J., and Neel, J.F., *A Clinical, Pathological and General Study of Multiple Neurofibromatosis*, Charles C. Thomas, Springfield, Ill., 1956.

'Death of the Elephant Man', report in the *British Medical Journal*, vol. I, 10 April 1890, pp. 916-17.

'Death of the Elephant Man', report on inquest in *The Times*, 16 April 1890.

Eaton, Colin, 'Freak Found Refuge on Northants Farm', *Northants Post*, 15 November 1980.

' "Elephant Man", The', report in the *British Medical Journal*, vol. II, 11 December 1886, pp. 1188-9.

Elephant Man, The, pamphlet amplified from an account published in the *British Medical Journal*, John Bale & Sons, London, 1888.

'Elephant Man, The', anonymous article in the *Illustrated Leicester Chronicle*, 27 December 1930.

Entract, J.P., 'The Elephant Man's Pied à Terre', *London Hospital Gazette*, vol. LXXIII, no. 2, May 1970.

Fienman, Norman L., and Yakovac, William C., 'Neurofibromatosis in Childhood', *Journal of Pediatrics*, vol. 76, no. 3, March 1970, pp. 339–46.

Flower, Sir Newman, *Just As It Happened*, Cassell, London, 1950.

Gomm, F.C. Carr, 'Death of the Elephant Man', letter to *The Times*, 16 April 1890.

Gomm, F.C. Carr, 'The Elephant Man', letter of appeal in *The Times*, 4 December 1886.

Grenfell, Sir Wilfred, *A Labrador Doctor*, revised popular edition, Hodder & Stoughton, London, 1929.

Halsted, D.G., *A Doctor in the Nineties*, Johnson, London, 1959.

Kendal, Madge, *Dame Madge Kendal by Herself*, John Murray, London, 1933.

Merrick, Joseph Carey, *The Autobiography of Joseph Carey Merrick*, Leicester, n.d.

Minutes of the London Hospital House Committee, 7 December 1886; 14 December 1886; 15 April 1890.

Montagu, Ashley, *The Elephant Man: A Study in Human Dignity*, Allison & Busby, London, 1972; Outerbridge & Dienstfrey, New York, 1971.

Norman, Tom, 'This is Tom Norman: Sixty-five Years a Showman and Auctioneer', unpublished MS. in possession of the Norman family.

Norman, Tom, letter of self-justification in the *World's Fair*, 24 February 1923.

Poole, E.F., *The Story of Byfield*, Archer & Goodman, Northampton, 1930; this repeats an article, 'The Romance of Redhill Wood', *Northampton County Magazine*, vol. 1, 1928, pp. 292–3.

Reed, Nicholas, 'The Mystery of Lot 583', *World Medicine*, 29 November 1980.

Reports of the first meeting of the Pathological Society of London to consider the case of the Elephant Man, *British Medical Journal*, vol. II, 6 December 1884, p. 1140; *Lancet*, vol. II, 6 December 1884, p. 1000; of the second meeting, *British Medical Journal*, vol. I, 21 March 1885, p. 595; *Lancet*, vol. I, 21 March 1885, pp. 1188–9.

Reviews of *The Elephant Man and Other Reminiscences* by Sir Frederick

Treves, *British Medical Journal*, vol. I, 17 March 1923, p. 335; *Lancet*, vol. I, 17 March 1923, pp. 547-8; *World's Fair*, 10 February 1923.

Somerset, Lady Geraldine, 'Private Journal of the Duchess of Cambridge', MS. diary in the Royal Archives, Windsor Castle Library.

Treves, Frederick, 'A Case of Congenital Deformity', *Transactions of the Pathological Society of London*, vol. XXXVI, 1885, pp. 494-8.

Treves, Sir Frederick, *The Elephant Man and Other Reminiscences*, Cassell, London, 1923.

Weber, F. Parkes, 'Cutaneous Pigmentation as an Incomplete Form of Recklinghausen's Disease, with Remarks on the Classification of Incomplete Forms of Recklinghausen's Disease', *British Journal of Dermatology*, vol. 21, 1949, pp. 49-51.

Weber, F. Parkes, *Further Rare Diseases and Debatable Subjects*, Staples Press, London, 1949.

Weber, F. Parkes, 'Periosteal Neurofibromatosis, with a Short Consideration of the Whole Subject of Neurofibromatosis', *Quarterly Journal of Medicine*, vol. 23, 1930, p. 151.

Wilson, S.A. Kinnier, *Neurology*, vol. 2, Arnold, London, 1940.

*

The story of Joseph Merrick in Treves's version provided the inspiration for the play by Bernard Pomerance, *The Elephant Man*, first produced at the Hampstead Theatre, London, in 1977, and later on Broadway and at the National Theatre in London; text published by Faber & Faber, London, 1980. Treves's story was, as well, the starting point for a film also called *The Elephant Man* (directed by David Lynch, starring John Hurt) which was released in 1980.

2. SELECTED LIST OF OTHER WORKS CONSULTED

'A Palace of Varieties for Leicester', *Nottingham Journal*, 3 September 1883.

Altick, Richard, *The Shows of London*, Belknap Press of Harvard University Press, 1978.

Cullen, Tom, *The Times and Crimes of Jack the Ripper* (originally entitled *Autumn of Terror*), Fontana, London, 1966.

Dallas, Duncan, *The Travelling People*, Macmillan, London, 1971.

Ellis, Colin D.B., *History in Leicester*, 2nd edition, City of Leicester Information Department, 1969.

Ellis, I.C., *Nineteenth Century Leicester*, Leicester, n.d.

Evans, Bergen, *The Natural History of Nonsense*, Michael Joseph, London, 1947.

Frost, Thomas, *The Old Showmen and the Old London Fairs*, Tinsley Brothers, London, 1874.

Hardwicke, Sir Cedric, *A Victorian in Orbit*, Methuen, London, 1961.

Hardy, Florence Emily, *The Life of Thomas Hardy, 1840–1928*, Macmillan, London, 1962.

Hone, William, 'The Editor's Visits to Claude Amboise Seurat', 26 July 1825; 'Visit to Bartholomew Fair', 5 September 1825; *The Every-day Book*, new edition, vol. 1, Thomas Tegg, London, 1841.

'Mr Sam Torr', *Music Hall*, 23 February 1889.

Morley, Henry, *Memoirs of Bartholomew Fair*, new edition, Chatto & Windus, London, 1880.

Obituary notices of Sir Frederick Treves: *British Medical Journal*, vol. II, 15 December 1923, pp. 1185–9; *Lancet*, vol. II, 15 December 1923, p. 1325; *The Times*, 10 December 1923.

Porter, Enid, *Cambridgeshire Customs and Folklore*, Routledge & Kegan Paul, London, 1969.

Porter, Enid, *The Folklore of East Anglia*, Batsford, London, 1974.

Reviews of the pantomime, *The Babes in the Wood*: *Illustrated London News*, 7 January 1888; *Punch*, 7 January 1888.

'Tom Norman', *The Era*, 26 October 1901.

Torr, Clara, MS. diary in possession of the Torr family.

Treves, Sir Frederick, *Highways and Byways in Dorset*, Macmillan, London, 1906.

Treves, Sir Frederick, *The Other Side of the Lantern*, Cassell, London, 1905.

Tyrwhitt-Drake, Sir Garrard, *The English Circus and Fairground*, Methuen, London, 1946.

Viski, Károly, *Hungarian Peasant Customs*, 2nd edition, George Vajnu, Budapest, 1937.

Wilson, A.E., *Christmas Pantomime*, Allen & Unwin, London, 1934.

INDEX

(*Figures in italic indicate a related illustration*)

The True History of the Elephant Man tells of the life of one man who suffered from neurofibromatosis. Joseph Merrick's may well be the most severe case ever recorded, but a proportion of the world's population carries the defective gene. There are probably about 20,000 people in the United Kingdom who do so, while the equivalent number for the United States, with its larger population, is probably in the region of 100,000. Many of these are likely to need varying degrees of medical help or counselling during the course of their lives.

Organizations have been set up to aid those who suffer from neurofibromatosis - to help to relieve the intense feelings of isolation from which Merrick also certainly suffered, and to act to make contact between sufferers and the medical profession in the hope of promoting a better understanding and awareness of the condition.

In the United Kingdom, anyone requiring further information should contact Trish Green, honorary secretary of LINK, 14 Willow Way, Sherfield on Lodden, Basingstoke, Hants. The corresponding organization in the United States is the National Neurofibromatosis Foundation Inc., 70 West 40th Street (4th Floor), New York, New York 10018.